DIABETES INDIA UPDATE 2025

DIABETES INDIA UPDATE 2025

Under the Aegis of Diabetes India

Editor-in-Chief

Shashank R Joshi

MD DM FICP FICN FRCP(London, Edinburgh, Glasgow) FACP

Past-President, API Past Dean, ICP, Mumbai, Maharashtra
Adjunct Faculty, Jaipur National University and JSS, Mysuru
Chief Advisor 2025
Immediate Past Chair IDF South East Asia
Consultant Endocrinologist, Lilavati, Sir HN Reliance and Joshi Clinic
Mumbai, Maharashtra, India

Executive Editor

Amit Gupta

MSc(Advancing Diabetes Care, BCU, UK) DNB(General Medicine) MNAMS
FACE FICP FRCP(Glasgow, Edinburgh) FACP FRSSDI F-Diab

Joint Secretary, Diabetes India Diabetologist and Metabolic Physican Medical Director
Centre for Diabetes Care
Greater Noida, Uttar Pradesh, India

Forewords

SR Aravind
Banshi Saboo

JAYPEE

JAYPEE BROTHERS MEDICAL PUBLISHERS

The Health Sciences Publisher

New Delhi | London

JAYPEE **Jaypee Brothers Medical Publishers (P) Ltd**

Headquarters
EMCA House
23/23-B, Ansari Road, Daryaganj
New Delhi 110 002, India
Landline: +91-11-23272143, +91-11-23272703
+91-11-23282021, +91-11-23245672
E-mail: jaypee@jaypeebrothers.com

Corporate Office
Jaypee Brothers Medical Publishers (P) Ltd.
4838/24, Ansari Road, Daryaganj
New Delhi 110 002, India
Phone: +91-11-43574357
Fax: +91-11-43574314
E-mail: jaypee@jaypeebrothers.com

Overseas Office
JP Medical Ltd.
83, Victoria Street, London
SW1H 0HW (UK)
Phone: +44-20 3170 8910
Fax: +44(0)20 3008 6180
E-mail: info@jpmedpub.com

Website: www.jaypeebrothers.com
Website: www.jaypeedigital.com

Inquiries for bulk sales may be solicited at: jaypee@jaypeebrothers.com

***Diabetes India Update 2025* / Shashank R Joshi**

First Edition: **2025**

ISBN: 978-93-6616-921-7

Printed at: Samrat Offset Pvt. Ltd.

Editorial Team for Diabetes Update by Diabetes India

Contributors

Author Name	Abstract No
Abha Gupta	63
Adriana Lapardhaja	70
Agam Vora	79
Ahmed Al-Sharefi	102
Ajoy Tewari	30
Akansha Singh	7
Akashkumar N Singh	86
Alka Chadha	62
Ameya Joshi	87
Ami Sanghvi	60
Ananda Basu	24, 54
Anant Nigam	80
Anil Kumar Virmani	3
Anju Seth	16
Antonio Ceriello	58
Anubha Srivastava	61, 84
Anurag Bajpai	18
Anushree Mehta	21
Aravind R Sosale	34
Aravinda J	49
Arvind Gupta	101
Ashish Kumar	82
Balaji Chidambaram	29
Balaji Jaganmohan	89
Bhavana Sosale	34
Bijay Patni	51
Brian Tomlinson	5, 6
Brij Mohan Makkar	8
Chandni Radhakrishnan	103
Collip Hall	81
Debashis Das	36
Debmalya Sanyal	83
Deepak Kumar Das	48
Evis Sinjari	70
Florian Toti	70
Hamid Ashraf	55
Hu Renming	43
Inge Van Boxalaer	17, 32
Jayant Agarwal	61, 84
Jaydip V Revale	40
Jibin Chi	11
JJ Mukherjee	77
Jothydev Kesavadev	23
Kalpana Jog	39
Kamlakar Tripathi	33
Kamlesh Khunti	85
Kannan Natarajan	68
Kiran Shah	35, 37
László Barkai	92
Lotika Purohit	93
Luftime Bruka	70
Madhu Pandey	14
Majken Brinkmann	13
Manisha Gupta	18
Manpreet Singh Brar	2
Marilda Hysa	70
Meena Srivastava	18
Meghna Gupta	2
Michel P Hermans	10, 91
Mikel Izquierdo	95, 96
Mohammed Yousuf Khan	90
Nebojsa M Lalic	12
Neeta Deshpande	9
Neeta Shah	31
NK Singh	97
P Popova	71
Parimal Swamy	20
Pranjali Shah	31
Praveen Gangadhara	59
Priya Phatak	66
Rajeev Chawla	74
Rakesh M Parikh	78
Ranjit Unnikrishnan	38
Raveendran AV	76
Ripun Borpuzari	1
Rishi Shukla	18
Rita Basu	42, 94
Ritu Johari	19, 31
RM Anjana	4
Robert A Vigersky	25, 26
Rosamma Joseph	103
Rukiya Shaikh	31
S Sengupta	100
Sahana V Gowda	34

Author Name	Abstract No
Sambit Das	41
Sandeep Rai	73
Sandeep Suri	67
Sangeeta Shukla	18
Sanket Pendsey	53
Saritha Kakani	64
Saurabh Mishra	18
Shambo Samrat Samajdar	44
Sheenam Gupta	41
Smita Shah	56

Author Name	Abstract No
Srikanth Narayana	34
Stephen Greene	27
Sudhir Chandra Jha	72
Swari Srivastava	65
Tatjana Milenkovic	69
Tejas Shah	28
Unnati Maniar	15
Usha Sharma	34
V Mohan	45, 75
Veer Bahadur Singh	99

Author Name	Abstract No
Vinod Kumar	57
Vinod Mittal	52
Vipul Chavda	98
Vitull K Gupta	2
Vivien Lim	50, 88
Wahid Khan	47
Warren Lee	22, 46, 81

Foreword

Diabetes is one of the most pressing global health challenges of our time, affecting millions of individuals and placing an ever-increasing burden on healthcare systems. The rapid evolution of research, technology, and clinical practices in diabetes management calls for continuous learning, collaboration, and innovation. It is in this spirit that DiabetesIndia 2025 brings together some of the finest minds in the field to share knowledge, discuss groundbreaking developments, and shape the future of diabetes care.

The *"Diabetes India Update 2025"* – Speaker Abstract Book is a reflection of the dedication and expertise of researchers, clinicians, and thought leaders who are committed to advancing diabetes science and improving patient outcomes. This collection of abstracts provides a glimpse into the latest research, emerging treatment modalities, and best practices that are transforming diabetes care on a global scale. It serves as a valuable resource for healthcare professionals, offering insights that will not only enhance clinical practice but also inspire new directions for future research.

We extend our deepest appreciation to all the distinguished faculty, researchers, and contributors who have made this publication possible. Their work embodies the collective effort to bridge the gap between research and real-world application, ensuring that patients receive the best possible care.

As you delve into the insights and discoveries presented in this book, we encourage you to engage in discussions, challenge conventional thinking, and explore opportunities for collaboration. The knowledge shared within these pages has the potential to drive meaningful advancements in diabetes management and empower healthcare professionals to make a lasting impact on the lives of those affected by this condition.

A special note of gratitude to Dr Shashank R Joshi and Dr Amit Gupta for their invaluable contributions to this initiative. Their guidance and expertise have played a crucial role in shaping the scientific program and this compendium.

We look forward to an enriching and stimulating exchange of ideas at DiabetesIndia 2025. May this conference serve as a platform for learning, networking, and fostering innovative solutions for the future of diabetes care.

Warm regards,

SR Aravind
President, DiabetesIndia

Banshi Saboo
Secretary, DiabetesIndia

Diabetes is one of the most pressing global health challenges of our time, affecting millions of individuals and placing an ever-increasing burden on healthcare systems. The rapid evolution of research, technology and clinical practices in diabetes management calls for continuous learning, collaboration, and innovation. It is in this spirit that [illegible]

[illegible] 2025 [illegible] and best [illegible] that will not only enhance clinical practice but also inspire new directions for [illegible]

[illegible]

Preface

Dear Colleagues and Friends,

It is with great enthusiasm that we present the *"Diabetes India Update 2025"* – Speaker Abstract Book, a compilation of the latest research, clinical advancements, and innovative discussions shaping the future of diabetes care. This book serves as a valuable resource, offering insights from leading experts dedicated to transforming the landscape of diabetes management.

DiabetesIndia 2025, the 15th World Congress, brings together over 200 renowned faculty members from across the globe, each contributing their expertise to enhance our understanding of diabetes. The conference embraces a multidisciplinary approach, covering a broad spectrum of topics, including pathophysiology, therapeutic strategies, glucose monitoring, emerging technologies, and the prevention and management of complications.

The abstracts in this book highlight the tireless commitment of researchers, clinicians, and scientists striving to improve patient care through evidence-based practice and innovation. These contributions are not just scientific discussions but stepping stones toward more effective diabetes prevention and treatment strategies.

We extend our heartfelt gratitude to the esteemed speakers, researchers, and contributors who have shared their work and knowledge. Their dedication to the field is instrumental in advancing our collective understanding of diabetes. We also appreciate the relentless efforts of the organizing committee, volunteers, and supporters who have made this conference possible.

As you explore the abstracts, we encourage you to engage with new ideas, challenge existing concepts, and cultivate collaborations that will drive meaningful change in diabetes care. Let this gathering be an opportunity for learning, networking, and inspiring one another toward a healthier future for our patients and communities.

We look forward to meaningful discussions, new friendships, and shared learning at DiabetesIndia 2025.

Warm regards,

Shashank R Joshi
Editor-in-Chief

Amit Gupta
Executive Editor

Acknowledgments

We extend our sincere gratitude to everyone who has contributed to the success of DiabetesIndia 2025 and the development of the *"Diabetes India Update 2025"* – Speaker Abstract Book. This compilation represents the collective efforts of researchers, clinicians, and experts who are dedicated to advancing diabetes care and improving patient outcomes.

We would like to express our heartfelt appreciation to all the distinguished faculty, speakers, and researchers for their invaluable contributions. Their work and insights have enriched this publication, making it a valuable resource for the medical community.

A special thanks go to the organizing committee, editorial team, and support staff who have worked tirelessly to ensure the smooth execution of this congress and the compilation of this book. Their dedication and commitment have been instrumental in bringing this project to fruition.

We are especially grateful to Dr Banshi Saboo, Dr SR Aravind, Dr Amit Gupta, and Dr Sanjay Reddy for their leadership, guidance, and continuous efforts in strengthening this platform for education and knowledge sharing. Their contributions have been essential in shaping the scientific program and ensuring a comprehensive approach to diabetes care.

We also extend our gratitude to Jaypee Brothers Medical Publishers (P) Ltd, New Delhi, India, for their invaluable support in publishing this book and ensuring its accessibility to a wider audience. Their collaboration has played a crucial role in bringing this edition to life.

Finally, we are grateful to the attendees and participants of DiabetesIndia 2025 for their enthusiasm and engagement. We hope that this book serves as a meaningful guide for continued learning and collaboration in the field of diabetes management.

Warm regards,

Sanjeev Pathak
Organizing Secretary, DiabetesIndia 2025

Manoj Chawla
Organizing Chairman, DiabetesIndia 2025

Contents

Section 1: Prediabetes and Risk Factors

Section 2: Type 1 Diabetes Management and Innovations

Section 3: Diagnostics and Biomarkers

Section 5: Clinical Approaches and Guidelines

Section 6: Complications and Comorbidities

COLOR PLATE

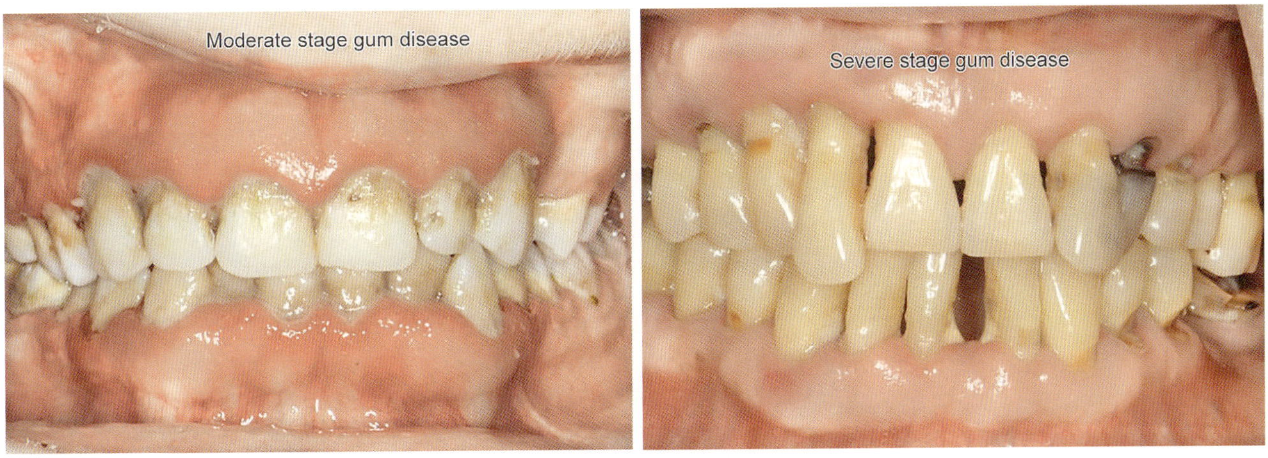

Abstract no 66: Should Periodontal Therapy be Standardized as Part of Diabetes Management Plans?

1
Section

Prediabetes and Risk Factors

1. Impact of Prediabetes on Women

Ripun Borpuzari

ABSTRACT

Prediabetes (PD) is on the rise globally. Studies around the world claim that the prevalence of PD is distinctively more in women that men at any age group, whereas men predominate in type 2 diabetes (T2D). This is parallel to the rising prevalence of obesity in women.

Impacts of PD in women depends on several factors like:

- Genetic and epigenetic factors:
    - Failure of X-inactivation of any obesogenic trait (e.g., *KDM5C* gene)
    - Exposure endocrine disruptors, etc., during germ cell development
- Altered effects of sex hormones (androgen excess) on adiposity and insulin sensitivity
- Unhealthy life style with hedonic eating behavior and physical inactivity during reproductive years
- And then, post-menopausal gradual loss of oestrogen protection.

Within the reproductive age, PD is detected almost always by showing impaired glucose tolerance (IGT), because of estrogen imparted hepatic insulin sensitivity resulting in normal fasting sugar. But when detected at or after menopause, there can be impaired fasting glucose (IFG) or mixed IFG and IGT depending on amount of IR on the muscular and adipose tissues and ongoing β cell dysfunction.

The overall impact of PD is summarised under the following headings.

- *Endocrine:* Progressing to T2D:
    - High life time risk of progressing to T2D;
    - PCOS (polycystic ovarian syndrome) having a bidirectional relation with PD.
- *Obesity/Overweight:* NFALD/MASLD
- *Reproductive health:* Gestational Diabetes, Reduced fecundability, adverse pregnancy outcomes.
- *Sexual health:* Effects on libido, reduced vaginal lubrication, etc.
- *Vascular Outcomes:* All macro- and microvascular complications with significant sex differences.
- *Bone Health:* Osteoporosis and fractures.
- *Mental Health:* Anxiety and depression as a result of central IR.
- *Cancers:* Is there any link?

Note: All relevant references are on the PPP.

2. Primary Prevention of Cardiometabolic Diseases in India

Vitull K Gupta, Meghna Gupta, Manpreet Singh Brar

ABSTRACT

Cardiometabolic diseases (CMDs) are a combination of cardiac and metabolic diseases and primary Prevention of CMDs involves understanding of the risk factors and measures to control those risk factors. Risk factors include non-modifiable risk factors like family history, race or ethnic background, age, gestational diabetes and modifiable risk factors include unhealthy diet, weight, physical activity, blood pressure, tobacco use, air pollution, prediabetes, dyslipidemia, polycystic ovary syndrome (PCOS), certain endocrine disorders and medications, stress, sleep disorders, education and income levels, metabolic syndrome and urbanisation. Primary Prevention of CMDs in India involves addressing the modifiable risk factors. Cultural and behavioural factors like unhealthy dietary habits, physical inactivity, tobacco and alcohol use are important. Socio-economic factors include income disparities, lack of awareness about healthy lifestyle choices and disease prevention and healthcare access especially in rural areas. Healthcare system factors include limited preventive care, insufficient resource allocation and shortage of trained healthcare professionals. Environmental factors include increasing pollution and rapid urbanization leading to lifestyle changes and increased stress. Policy and implementation are important factors which include weak implementation of policies related to tobacco, alcohol, and food industries and lack of effective public health initiatives. Burden of CMD risk factors is significant and is increasing in India. Various cultural, socio-economic and systemic challenges are critical for prevention of CMDs. Addressing these risk factors requires a multifaceted approach involving public health interventions, lifestyle changes, medical management, community initiatives, public health campaigns, healthcare system strengthening and promotion of healthy lifestyle behaviors from childhood. Implementing comprehensive strategies that target prevention, early detection, and management of CMDs is crucial for reducing their burden and prevention of CMDs in India.

3. Tackling the Menace of T2DM in 2025: What are the Key Issues?

Anil Kumar Virmani

ABSTRACT

There are five major issues:

1. Is it time to Focus on Prevention of T2DM?

   The prevalence of T2DM in India is about 10–11% and stabilized in most states, but the prevalence of Pre-Diabetes is >15%, which is very alarming and a volcano waiting to erupt. We should now prioritize our focus on Primary Prevention by Mass Awareness and Education Programs, Screening, Identifying and Risk-stratifying high-risk patients with Pre-Diabetes, and appropriate non-pharmacological and Pharmacological interventions, to modify risk factors like Obesity and Insulin Resistance. Moreover, we should also be focussing on Primordial Prevention by taking care of the maternal and Foetal health.

2. Why Individualisation of therapy is the key to success?
   Approach to a patient with diabetes will depend upon various factors in deciding the target HbA1c and the appropriate use of drugs with pleiotropic effects. All decisions should be patient-centred and based on shared decision making.
3. Why think holistically?
   Besides glycaemic control, it is very important to simultaneously target Obesity, Hypertension, Dyslipidaemia, Smoking and Alcohol Abuse, Sedentariness, Sleep disorders, Stress and emotional health.
4. What works and when?
   Intensive life-style modification should be rigorously enforced and reminded at every visit in all patients. Early stages of Diagnosis need intensive measures for strict glycaemic control, whereas long duration of diabetes with multiple co-morbidities may require more emphasis on use of cardio-renal protecting drugs.
5. Who takes the responsibility?
   The goals of treatment are to prevent complications and optimize Quality of Life. A multidisciplinary approach with a well-informed, motivated, and empowered patient are the keys to success in diabetes care.

4. Diabetes in Women: What is Different?

RM Anjana

ABSTRACT

Diabetes is growing in epidemic proportions in many countries including India resulting in a significant increase in morbidity and mortality. The Indian Council of Medical Research–India DIABetes (ICMR–INDIAB) study, the largest nationally representative epidemiological survey conducted in 113,043 adults aged ≥20 years (52,602-men and 60,441-women) reported an overall prevalence of diabetes and prediabetes to be 11.4% and 15.3% respectively, corresponding to 101 million people with diabetes and 136 million people with prediabetes in India. Although this study reported that diabetes prevalence is lower in women (10.7%) compared to men (12.1%), women face unique challenges compared to men. This study also reported that impaired fasting glucose prevalence was significantly higher among women (Women: 10.7% vs. Men: 9.4%) while impaired glucose tolerance among men (Women: 2.9% vs. Men: 3.7%). The study found that good glycemic and blood pressure control was achieved equally among both sexes in individuals with self-reported diabetes (36.0% and 49.0% respectively). Total and LDL cholesterol control was better among males, and triglyceride control was better among females. These differences may be due to gender disparities in access to and affordability of treatment, as well as potential differences in medication adherence and consistency. Furthermore, women reported less frequent self-monitoring, lower levels of physical activity, and reduced consumption of fruits and vegetables compared to men. Additionally, women with diabetes are more likely to experience complications such as neuropathy, peripheral vascular disease, depression, stress and anxiety, which can impact their ability to manage their condition effectively. Thus, early detection, proper management, and lifestyle interventions are crucial for preventing complications and improving outcomes for women with diabetes.

5. Management of Obesity to Prevent Atherosclerosis

Brian Tomlinson

ABSTRACT

Obesity promotes atherosclerosis through various mechanisms including dyslipidemia, hypertension, insulin resistance and inflammation. Weight loss by lifestyle intervention can reduce the risk of atherosclerosis but is often not very effective in the long term. Bariatric surgery is effective in reducing weight and atherosclerosis risk but is not always available and patients may not be willing to undergo it. The glucagon-like peptide-1 receptor agonists (GLP-1 RAs) were developed for the treatment of type 2 diabetes but some of the long-acting GLP-1 RAs, particularly liraglutide and semaglutide are very effective in reducing body weight and the associated cardiovascular risk factors. The dual glucose-dependent insulinotropic polypeptide (GIP) and GLP-1 RA, tirzepatide, has greater effects on some of the cardiovascular risk factors and may prove to be even more effective in reducing atherosclerotic cardiovascular disease (ASCVD) events than pure GLP-1 RAs. Other dual and triple agonists such as retatrutide in development may also prove very effective. The combination of cagrilintide with semaglutide, marketed as CagriSema, is a combination of semaglutide with the dual amylin and calcitonin receptor agonist, cagrilintide, and this may result in greater weight loss than either drug alone. Various other combinations are in development and whether these combinations will have advantages in reducing ASCVD events remains to be seen.

Sodium-glucose cotransporter-2 (SGLT-2) inhibitors also reduce body weight but to a lesser extent than GLP-1 RAs and they are not considered as treatments for obesity. Their benefits appear to be more related to heart failure and chronic kidney disease rather than ASCVD, but the combination with GLP-1 RAs may have additional cardiovascular benefits.

6. The Vexed Problem of Moderate Hypertriglyceridemia and Elevated Remnant Cholesterol

Brian Tomlinson

ABSTRACT

Hypertriglyceridemia is a heterogeneous condition with a polygenic background and major contributions from lifestyle, diet and other conditions, particularly diabetes and obesity. Moderate elevation of triglycerides in triglyceride-rich lipoproteins (TRLs) is an independent risk factor for cardiovascular disease (CVD), whereas severe hypertriglyceridemia (>10 mmol/L) is a risk factor for acute pancreatitis. Non-high-density lipoprotein (non-HDL) cholesterol incudes the remnant cholesterol carried in TRLs in addition to the cholesterol in low-density lipoprotein cholesterol (LDL-C) and is regarded as a secondary or alternative target for lipid treatment. Genetic studies showed that triglyceride-lowering genetic variants were associated with lower risk of CVD in proportion to the reduction in apoB and these studies have identified new therapeutic targets including angiopoietin-like protein 3 (ANGPTL3) and apolipoprotein C3 (apoC3).

Lifestyle and diet intervention is the essential first line management and it is important to try to optimize control of other conditions such as diabetes and obesity. Effective glycemic control will usually reduce triglyceride levels and some treatments for diabetes, particularly the glucagon-like peptide-1 receptor agonists (GLP-1 RAs), have additional benefits on lipid levels. Likewise, reduction of obesity with GLP-1 RAs can also improve plasma lipids. Fibrates are one of the most useful treatments for reducing triglycerides and they are usually effective in reducing severe elevations of triglycerides to safer levels, but their effects in reducing cardiovascular events have been variable. Certain omega-3 fatty acid treatments, particularly those which only contain eicosapentaenoic acid (EPA) such as icosapent ethyl, have proven benefits in reducing the risk of CVD in patients with moderate hypertriglyceridemia and these are recommended in current guidelines. Drugs in development targeting ApoC3 or ANGPTL3 may prove to be useful in this situation.

7. PCOS and Type 2 Diabetes: Breaking the Vicious Cycle

Akansha Singh

ABSTRACT

Polycystic ovary syndrome (PCOS) is a multisystem disorder usually seen in females who are in their reproductive age (15–49 years of age). People with PCOS have metabolic and endocrine abnormalities the most striking of them is the presence of Insulin resistance along with compensatory hyperinsulinemia.

Insulin resistance is thought to be due to post-binding abnormality with abnormal autophosphorylation of the beta sub-unit of insulin receptor and Insulin substrate-1. There is decrease in tyrosine phosphorylation and an increase in serine phosphorylation, which reduces insulin metabolism. PCOS also affects the function of beta cells of pancreas. Hence, Insulin resistance and beta cell dysfunction increases the risk of developing DM in women with PCOS.

The association of PCOS with increased T2D risk is relatively robust and thus should not be neglected in any woman with the syndrome. Despite the current heterogeneity of the data and the uncertainty regarding exact mechanisms regulating progression of dysglycemia in PCOS, there are several principles that the clinician should implement in everyday practice. First, diagnosis and follow-up of dysglycemia should preferably be based on OGTT values. Second, the non-linear development of T2D in PCOS in non-obese women highlights the importance of maintaining an optimal weight in all women suffering from the syndrome. Third, menopausal women with a history of PCOS in non-obese should be regularly evaluated since they may be at higher T2D risk, especially if they are obese. Fourth, a well-balanced diet coupled with regular exercise constitutes the most appropriate approach in every patient with PCOS. Metformin administration might ameliorate the biochemical and hormonal profile in PCOS and may be considered in patients in whom prior measures have failed to improve metabolic and ovulatory dysfunction. The use of Pioglitazone, GLP-1-RAs, and/or MHT may be of value in selected cases.

8. The Role of New Generation Antiobesity Medicines in Preventing Diabetes

Brij Mohan Makkar

ABSTRACT

Introduction

Prevalence of obesity is rising globally and it is the key driver for increasing prevalence of type 2 diabetes. There is a strong association between obesity, especially central obesity, and increased risk of type 2 diabetes. Studies have shown that a rise in obesity prevalence in a population is paralleled by rising prevalence of type 2 diabetes. Therefore, it is logical to address obesity to reduce the risk of type 2 diabetes.

Studies with lifestyle interventions for prevention of diabetes, namely DPS, DPP, Da Qing study, have shown that even a modest weight reduction can lead to significant lowering of risk for developing type 2 diabetes.

This has also been shown with weight loss medications. One of the earliest studies to show the impact of weight loss medications on diabetes prevention was Xendos study showing a 37% reduction in the risk of developing type 2 diabetes in persons with obesity treated with orlistat over a 4 year period. Similarly, Lorcaserin in Bloom and Blossom studies showed a significant reduction in the risk of progession to diabetes.

Earliest evidence for the role of GLP-1 RAs in prevention of diabetes was documented in SCALE PREDIABETES study showing significant reduction in the risk of diabetes in people with obesity treated with injection liraglutide 3 mg. Similar observations have been made with newer, more potent GLP-1 RA semaglutide showing more than 60% reduction in the risk of developing diabetes. In view of emerging evidence, it is quite likely that antiobesity medications will play a significant role in reducing the risk of developing type 2 diabetes.

9. How to Deliver Obesity Care in Clinical Practice

Neeta Deshpande

ABSTRACT

Introduction: This abstract addresses the critical need for structured obesity management in clinical practice, particularly within the Indian context. Current guidelines advocate for a move beyond a solely BMI-centric approach towards a more comprehensive, complication-centered strategy.

The proposed algorithm: A four-step process for obesity management is outlined. Step 1 involves anthropometric evaluation, assessing BMI, waist circumference, and other parameters, while acknowledging the limitations of relying on BMI alone. Step 2 focuses on clinical evaluation, including laboratory tests for comorbidities and impacts such as metabolic conditions, cardiovascular risk, and psychological well-being. Step 3 entails risk stratification and management, with interventions ranging from lifestyle modifications to pharmacotherapy and bariatric surgery, guided by the severity of the condition. Finally, Step 4 emphasizes follow-up to monitor progress and adjust the treatment plan as necessary.

Step 1 Anthropometric evaluation

Assess BMI and waist circumference
(Additional parameters: Hip circumference and waist-to-height ratio)

Step 2 Clinical evaluation (including laboratory tests) for comorbidities and impacts

- Evaluate complications and consequences (including comorbidities and physiological and psychological impacts)
- Endocrine evaluation tests (if applicable/necessary in the particular case)
- Socioeconomic status

Step 3 Risk stratification and management

As per step 1 findings (anthropometric evaluation)

BMI <23 kg/m^2 and waist circumference ≤ 80 cm in women, ≤ 90 cm in men
↓
Prevent weight gain → Heathy meal, physical activity, and health education

BMI ≥ 23 kg/m^2 and/or waist circumference >80 cm in women, >90 cm in men
↓
Perform EOSS staging* considering the step 2 findings (clinical evaluation)
↓

Complications	Stage 0	Stage 1	Stage 2	Stage 3	Stage 4
Medical	No risk factor	Pre-clinical	Comorbidity	End-organ damage	End stage
Psychological	Absent	Mild	Moderate	Severe	Very severe
Functional	Absent	Mild	Moderate	Severe	Very severe

Management modality as per staging

Stage 0 | Stage 1 | Stage 2 | Stage 3 | Stage 4

Lifestyle modifications (Stage 0–4)
- Calorie restriction, physical activity, and behavioral therapy
- For stage 1, pharmacotherapy can be considered if BMI ≥ 27 kg/m^2 and lifestyle interventions alone are not effective

Pharmacotherapy (BMI ≥ 25 kg/m^2) (Stage 2–4)
- Once weekly injectable semaglutide 2.4 mg**/tablet orlistat 120 mg
- For stage 2, bariatric surgery may be considered if BMI ≥ 32.5 kg/m^2 on a case-to-case basis if lifestyle interventions and pharmacotherapy are not effective

Bariatric surgery if BMI ≥ 32.5 kg/m^2 (Stage 3–4)

Step 4 **Follow-up**

- Plan the follow-up dates/periods–2/3/6 months and set targets to be evaluated
- Modify treatment plan (if needed)

*Refer to figure 1 for more details on EOSS staging: **Semaglutide 2.4 mg has been approved for obesity management, but not yet available in the Indian market

Results: The algorithm recommends the combined use of BMI and waist circumference for better identification of at-risk individuals. It also emphasizes ethnic-specific cutoffs for these measures. The algorithm categorizes risk based on the presence and severity of complications, guiding treatment intensity. Lifestyle modifications, including diet and exercise, are the first line of treatment, while pharmacotherapy, is considered for those with a BMI over 25 kg/m^2 with comorbidities or over 27 kg/m^2. Bariatric surgery is an option for patients with a BMI of 32 kg/m^2 or higher, or with certain comorbidities and a BMI above 27.5 kg/m^2. A multidisciplinary team approach is recommended, involving physicians, dietitians, physiotherapists, psychologists, and other specialists.

Conclusion: Implementing a structured algorithm for obesity management will help individualize treatment plans, optimize patient outcomes, and improve the benefit-risk ratio and cost-effectiveness of interventions. This approach emphasizes the importance of lifestyle modifications, pharmacotherapy, and surgery when indicated.

REFERENCE

1. Deshpande NR, Kapoor N, Dalal JJ, Palshetkar N, Shah S, Makkar BM, Wasir J, Selvan C. Consensus on Current Landscape and Treatment Trends of Obesity in India for Primary Care Physicians. J Assoc Physicians India. 2023;71(10):69-77.

10. The Intersection of Diabetes, Atherosclerosis, and Inflammation: New Therapeutic Targets

Michel P Hermans

ABSTRACT

Atherosclerotic/thrombotic cardiovascular disease (ASCVD – atherosclerosis) is a lipid-driven chronic inflammatory disease of the arteries, in which intimal deposition of cholesterol from LDLs and triglycerides-rich lipoproteins (TRL) remnants is not compensated by removal through HDL-driven reverse cholesterol transport. ASCVD is also a systemic or local inflammation-driven process, characterized by dysadipokinemia and raised CRP. Many CV and cardiometabolic risk factors, often at play in type 2 diabetes (T2D), are linked to endothelial damage, the preclinical stage of ASCVD. Inflammatory cytokines, including those arising from excess or hypoxic adipose tissue, are involved in T2DM onset, by fostering B-cell function loss and insulin resistance. They also promote LDL oxidation and ASCVD, whereas chronic hyperglycemia is associated with endothelial dysfunction, oxidative stress, and chronic inflammation, poorly-controlled T2D reinforcing the detrimental effects of obesity. Besides smoking cessation, BP- and lipid-lowering and anti-thrombotic drugs, anti-inflammatory therapies are increasingly considered as promising component of the therapeutic arsenal against ASCVD. Both colchicine, a tubulin polymerization inhibitor and canakinumab, an anti-interleukin-1β antibody SC (CANTOS trial) have demonstrated efficacy in reducing inflammation linked to ASCVD and adverse CV outcomes. Potential anti-atherosclerotic downstream modulation of proinflammatory cascade with IL-6 receptor antagonist tocilizumab is under investigation.

REFERENCES

1. Donath MY, Shoelson SE. Type 2 diabetes as an inflammatory disease. Nat Rev Immunol. 2011;11(2):98-107.
2. Calle MC, Fernandez ML. Inflammation and type 2 diabetes. Diabetes Metab. 2012;38(3):183-91.
3. Golia E, Limongelli G, Natale F, et al. Inflammation and cardiovascular disease: from pathogenesis to therapeutic target. Curr Atheroscler Rep. 2014;16:435.
4. d'Aiello A, Filomia S, Brecciaroli M, Sanna T, Pedicino D, Liuzzo G. Targeting inflammatory pathways in atherosclerosis: exploring new opportunities for treatment. Curr Atheroscler Rep. 2024;26(12):707-19.
5. Ait-Oufella H, Libby P. Inflammation and Atherosclerosis: Prospects for Clinical Trials. Arterioscler Thromb Vasc Biol. 2024;44(9):1899-905.

11. The Perfect Storm in Diabetes: How Insulin, Glucagon, and Dietary Fallacies Fuel a Global Epidemic

Jibin Chi

ABSTRACT

On May 3, 1922, Dr Macleod announced the discovery of insulin in a report titled "The Effects Generated on Diabetes by Extracts of Pancreas." This marked the first use of the term "insulin." In the same year, two researchers identified another pancreatic extract that raised blood glucose levels. Named glucagon (GLUCose-AGONist), it was initially dismissed as a "toxic fraction" associated with hyperglycemia and even death. While insulin was hailed as a medical breakthrough, earning Nobel recognition, glucagon remained overlooked for decades. The discovery of insulin also established the first partnership among academia, physicians, and the pharmaceutical industry, redefining diabetes as a condition of insufficient insulin secretion or impaired insulin action.

One hundred years after insulin's discovery, it is staggering how a once-rare disease has become a catastrophic global epidemic. Numerous studies have since unveiled the complex interplay between insulin and glucagon, mediated by incretin hormones and dietary influences. Despite this growing body of evidence, century-old misconceptions about insulin, glucagon, and diabetes have obstructed progress in challenging the foundations of diabetes science.

To address this reality, a new disruptive theory that aims to identify the "Perfect Storm in Diabetes" is being put forward. This theory spotlights the "three musketeers"—insulin, glucagon, and healthy diets—which were historically regarded as the cornerstones of diabetes science. Misconceptions and practices associated with these key elements have fueled a global health crisis that extends far beyond diabetes.

The theory initiates and proposes a unified disease model linking all chronic metabolic disorders, including liver diseases and cancer. It calls for a critical re-evaluation of diabetes science and clinical guidelines, offering a path to combat this mounting health crisis and save lives.

12. Diabetes Treatment, Obesity and Cardiovascular Disease: An Everchanging Puzzle

Nebojsa M Lalic

ABSTRACT

The prevalence of obesity worldwide has increased in recent decades and represents a global public health crisis that contributes to poor health outcomes. Obesity is a major risk factor for both diabetes and cardiovascular diseases (CVD) leading to insulin resistance and increased cardiovascular impairments. On the other hand, diabetes and obesity were found to be independently associated with adverse CV risk factors and major CV events. When combined, their risks were additive. Both obesity and diabetes are linked to CVD via multiple direct and indirect pathophysiological mechanisms, i.e., they contribute to the development of insulin resistance, endothelial dysfunction, increased vascular resistance, low-grade inflammation and prothrombotic state, which promote atherosclerosis. Effective diabetes treatment plays a crucial role in managing obesity and blood glucose levels and preventing the complications, including heart disease. Lifestyle interventions, such as dietary modifications and increased physical activity, are essential in mitigating these risks. Evidences indicate that intentional weight loss (more than 10%) lowers CVD risk among people with overweight/ obesity. Pharmacological approaches, including the use of anti-diabetic medications with weight management ability, offer additional support in achieving optimal health outcomes. Furthermore, recent advancements in understanding the pathophysiological links between these conditions emphasize the importance of an integrated management strategy that addresses weight control, blood glucose regulation, and cardiovascular health. New medicines for weight loss, specifically incretin-based therapies, are showing significant risk reduction for CV death, myocardial infarction (MI) and stroke in individuals with diabetes and obesity. Data obtained in previous years in numerous CV outcome studies have led to a paradigm shift in the treatment of type 2 diabetes and all current guidelines prioritize GLP-1 RA in specific patient populations. Moreover, new data have demonstrated a synergistic effect when lifestyle changes and GLP-1 RAs were used simultaneously on the prevention of CVD in obese diabetic patients.

13. Intermittent Fasting and Ketogenic Diets in Type 2 Diabetes: Evidence and Clinical Insights

Majken Brinkmann

ABSTRACT

Dietary strategies such as intermittent fasting (IF) and ketogenic diets (KD) are emerging as potential complementary approaches to managing Type 2 diabetes. While early research indicates promising results, the evidence remains limited, and long-term effects are still under investigation. This presentation reviews key findings from Danish and global studies and reflects on clinical observations.

A Danish pilot study demonstrated that a 10-hour eating window over 12 weeks led to reductions in HbA1c (4 mmol/mol) and weight loss (2 kg), alongside improved sleep and energy levels. The ongoing RESET2 study builds on these findings by investigating the long-term metabolic effects of time-restricted eating. Systematic reviews and meta-analyses suggest that KD can support glycemic control, including a reduction in HbA1c (up to 1%), and promote weight loss, though individual variability and long-term safety considerations remain important.

Drawing on 15 years of clinical experience, this session discusses the practical and theoretical aspects of integrating these dietary strategies into Type 2 diabetes care. Emphasis is placed on the need for further robust research and alignment with national dietary guidelines to ensure safe and effective implementation.

Keywords: Intermittent Fasting, Ketogenic Diet, Type 2 Diabetes, HbA1c, RESET2 Study, Clinical Applications

Topic: Diabetes and Varied Diets: Intermittent Fasting, Ketogenic Diets and Holiday Fasting

14. NAFLD and Cardiovascular Disease Risk

Madhu Pandey

ABSTRACT

Background: Non-alcoholic fatty liver disease (NAFLD) affects 25–30% of the global population and is increasingly recognized as a significant contributor to cardiovascular disease (CVD). NAFLD ranges from simple liver fat accumulation to more severe forms like nonalcoholic steatohepatitis (NASH), fibrosis, and cirrhosis. It is closely associated with metabolic syndrome, insulin resistance, Type 2 diabetes, dyslipidemia, and systemic inflammation, all of which heighten CVD risk. Emerging evidence suggests that NAFLD contributes independently to endothelial dysfunction, atherosclerosis, and arterial stiffness, positioning it as an independent risk factor for coronary artery disease, heart failure, and arrhythmias. Advanced liver fibrosis correlates with higher cardiovascular morbidity and mortality, emphasizing the importance of fibrosis staging.

Objectives: This abstract explores the relationship between NAFLD and CVD risk, examining shared pathophysiological mechanisms, clinical implications, and management strategies.

Key Findings:

- *Pathophysiological link*: NAFLD shares common risk factors with CVD, including obesity, insulin resistance, hypertension, and dyslipidemia. Systemic inflammation, oxidative stress, and endothelial dysfunction in NAFLD contribute to accelerated atherosclerosis and higher cardiovascular event risk.
- *Cardiovascular Manifestations*: NAFLD patients are at an increased risk for coronary artery disease, arterial stiffness, heart failure (especially HFpEF), and arrhythmias like atrial fibrillation.
- *Independent Risk Markers*: Liver fat is a significant predictor of cardiovascular risk, even without traditional metabolic factors.
- *Diagnostic Challenges*: Early identification requires a combination of imaging, biomarkers, and risk stratification tools.

Management Approaches: Lifestyle changes (weight loss, diet, physical activity) are crucial. Emerging pharmacotherapies, such as GLP-1 receptor agonists and SGLT-2 inhibitors, show promise for addressing both NAFLD and CVD risk factors.

Conclusion: NAFLD is a multisystem disorder with significant cardiovascular implications. Interdisciplinary management is essential for reducing hepatic and cardiovascular complications. Future research should focus on the bidirectional relationship and developing targeted therapies.

15. Effectiveness of MNT: Types of Diet for Treating Patients with Diabetes and Dyslipidemia

Unnati Maniar

ABSTRACT

Background: Diabetes is a rising public health concern in India, specially the cases of Type 2 Diabetes has been rapidly increasing. The comorbidities associated with diabetes is also increase one of which is dyslipidaemia. Dyslipidemia are characterized by abnormal concentrations of circulating lipids, increasing the risk of atherosclerosis and other serious conditions. Hyperinsulinemia is associated with low HDL cholesterol levels and hypertriglyceridemia in patient with diabetes. Most patients with diabetes are on statin therapy and various other medicines like fibrates or niacin or ezetimibe. But medication alone is not the only factor, dietary and lifestyle factors like excise are crucially important. Many researches show improvement in lipid levels as well as glucose control in patients following medication and medical nutrition therapy in combination. This paper is focused on Nutrition interventions for addressing concurrent elevations in LDL-C and TG include a combination of the strategies described for lowering LDL-C and TG as well as remission of type 2 diabetes.

Objective: To study the effect of different diet plans in patient with diabetes and dyslipidemia.

Inclusion Criteria: Type 2 DM, Continue on same medication for at least 3-month, Age: 18-55 years

Exclusion Criteria: Type 1 DM, Other types of Diabetes, recently changed medication.

Method: A retrospective interventional study was conducted with 40 participants diagnosed with type 2 diabetes and dyslipidemia. Subjects were enrolled in a 12-week structured nutritional therapy program involving diet counseling, meal planning, and monitoring by certified dietitians. Primary outcomes included changes in HbA1c, fasting blood glucose, postprandial blood glucose, total cholesterol, LDL, HDL, and triglyceride levels. Secondary outcomes focused on adherence and patient satisfaction. Two groups were formed, Group 1 followed a Routine Diabetes Diet (RDD) where total calorie intake was between 1,500–1,600 kcal, carbohydrate 50–55% (188–220 g/day), proteins: 15–20% (56–80 g/day), Fats: 25–30% (42–53 g/day) and the other group followed a Low Calorie Diet (LCD) with 1,100–1,200 kcal, Carbohydrates: 40–45% (120–146 g/day), Proteins: 20–25% (60–81 g/day), Fats: 30–35% (40–50 g/day) and fibre around 20–25 g/day was kept same for both the groups.

Result: Finding show that the group following LCD has better results than the group following RDD. The low-calorie diet improved the blood glucose level and lipid profile.

Conclusion: Our study suggests that a low-carbohydrate diet (LCD) yields better results compared to a regular diabetic diet (RDD). However, four participants were unable to adhere to the LCD due to its stricter regimen. Still more research is required to know about the sustainability and various other factors like physical activity and co-morbities need to be considered to show a better result.

REFERENCES

1. Feingold KR. Dyslipidemia in Patients with Diabetes. Endotext - NCBI Bookshelf. 2023. https://www.ncbi.nlm.nih.gov/books/NBK305900/
2. Zhang Y, Wang J, Li X. Nutritional therapy in the management of diabetes and dyslipidemia: A comprehensive review. J Nutr Biochem. 2003;105:108123.
3. Kirkpatrick CF, Sikand G, Petersen KS, et al. Nutrition interventions for adults with dyslipidemia: A clinical perspective from the National Lipid Association. J Clin Lipidol. 2023;17(4):428-51.

2
Section

Type 1 Diabetes Management and Innovations

16. 30 Years after DCCT: Transforming T1D Care in India

Anju Seth

ABSTRACT

India has the world's highest number of children and adolescents suffering from T1D. However, in face of huge pandemic of T2D in India, problems faced by children with T1D are often overlooked. There are many challenges to care of these children, including access to quality healthcare, management complexity, financial constraints, psychological impact and finally, transition to adult care.

T1D care involves management of emergencies like DKA, and provision of long-term ambulatory care. The latter has multiple components including assessment of glycemic control and individualized adjustment in insulin therapy, growth monitoring, care of intercurrent sickness, screening for comorbidities and complications, addressing psycho-social needs and issues of concern, diabetes education and introduction to new technology. It thus requires a team effort with involvement of experienced pediatrician/pediatric endocrinologist, Pediatric intensive care services, Nurse/Diabetes Educator, nutritionist, social worker and other specialists as required. This optimum care is currently available only at Medical colleges and associated hospitals and large Private hospitals in big cities. The costs are high and not within the reach of every needy person.

Government organisations like CGHS, ESI, Railways provide insulins and syringes to their beneficiaries. However, availability of glucometer, strips, CGMS devices and insulin pump is patchy and no clear guidelines regarding their prescription exists. CGHS has in recent times, issued guidelines regarding prescription of basic insulin pump to its beneficiaries. For the vast majority of affected persons, there is no formal system in place for uninterrupted provision of necessary supplies and optimum long-term care. A few State Governments, Institutes, NGOs and pharmaceutical companies provide support at their initiative to a variable extent.

There is an urgent need for providing comprehensive T1D care at the community level. At the very least, free continuous supply of insulins, injecting devices, periodic monitoring of glycemic control and responsive adjustment in insulin dose/lifestyle, complication screening and diabetes education to optimize outcome are needed.

17. Demystifying DIY Pancreas Systems: A Guide for Beginners

Inge Van Boxalaer

ABSTRACT

Automated Insulin Delivery (AID) systems have emerged as a transformative tool for managing insulin delivery in individuals with type 1 diabetes and insulin-deficient diabetes. Among these, open-source AID systems have gained prominence due to their proven safety, efficacy, and accessibility. These systems, free to download and implement, offer a cost-effective alternative to commercial systems, particularly for patients in resource-limited settings. However, the widespread adoption of open-source AID systems presents unique challenges, particularly the need for healthcare providers (HCPs) to support and educate patients effectively.

This presentation addresses the educational gap surrounding open-source AID systems by providing a comprehensive overview tailored for beginners. It introduces the most commonly used open-source systems, such as AndroidAPS and DIY Loop, alongside practical instructions on their setup and use. Participants will gain insights into the hardware and software components required, including continuous glucose monitors (CGMs), insulin pumps, and bridging devices.

Additionally, the presentation emphasizes the critical role of HCPs in supporting patients transitioning to open-source systems. Drawing on international consensus guidelines, it outlines best practices for educating patients about the benefits, limitations, and practical implementation of these systems. The session also highlights freely available, accredited, video-based e-learning modules designed to equip HCPs with the necessary knowledge and skills.

By bridging the knowledge gap, this session aims to empower HCPs and patients, enhancing the quality of diabetes care globally. Attendees will leave equipped to navigate the evolving landscape of open-source AID systems, promoting informed patient autonomy and improved glycemic control. This collaborative approach to diabetes management underscores the potential of open-source AID systems to revolutionize care and reduce the global burden of diabetes.

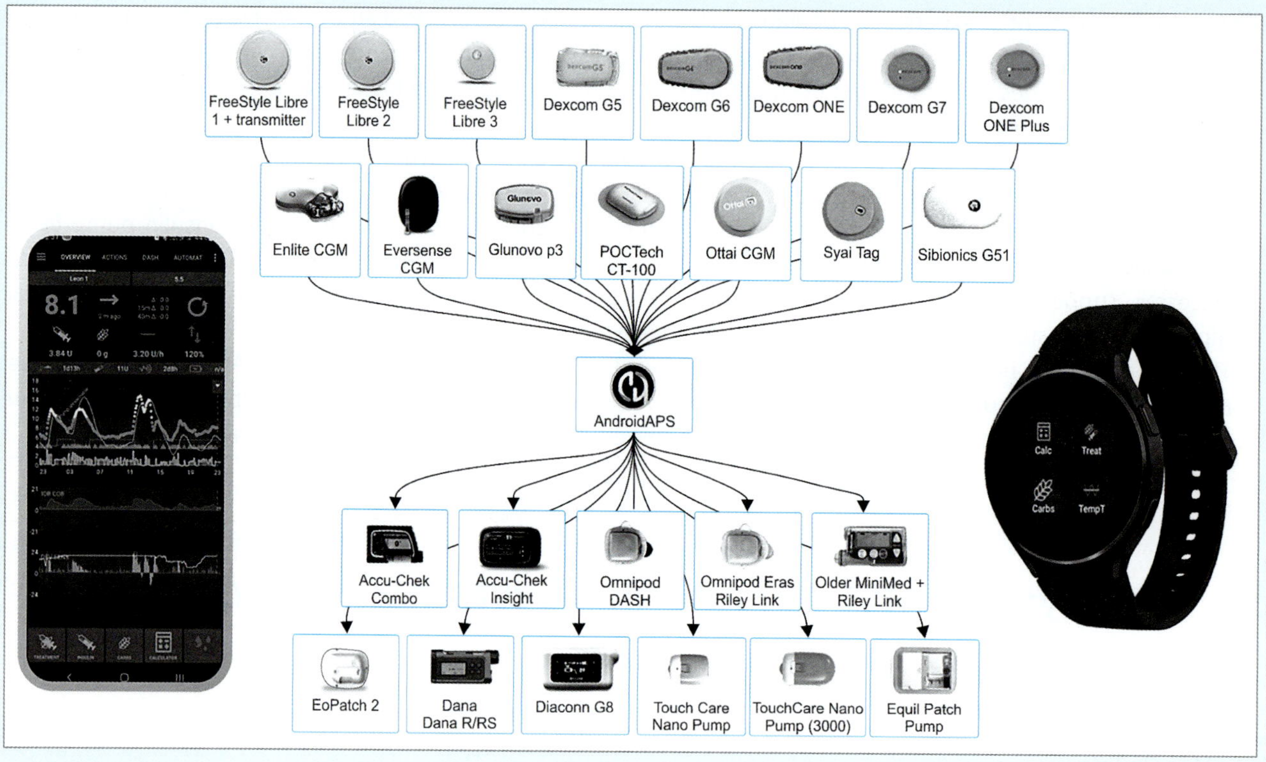

Disclosure: The author used GPT-4o for copywriting during abstract preparation, reviewed and edited the content, and takes full responsibility for the final publication.

18. Acceptance to Insulin Pump Therapy Increases with Group Installation and Group Education

Saurabh Mishra, Rishi Shukla, Anurag Bajpai, Manisha Gupta, Sangeeta Shukla, Meena Srivastava

ABSTRACT

Background: Pump Initiation in non government approved setting is always a problem. We took this entirely different initiative of pump education and initiation in T1DM children. For the first time in the history of pump we used this method.

AIM: To study the impact of Insulin Pump initiation in group education program.

Material and Methods: A 3 hours insulin pump training workshop was organized for patients to educate them about insulin pump. In this programme T1DM and next to the kin were involved. In this training programme 30 patients were enrolled. These patients were taught about insulin pump and hands on experience were done. Out of 30 patients 12 patients were ready to get insulin pump installed, 4 patients postponed the installation due to lack of affordability. A group installation of insulin pump was done in 8 patients at a time and they were allowed to share their experiences about pump. A follow up study of these 8 patients continued and we evaluated the level of satisfaction amongst the group installation group versus individual installation group from our past records.

Results	Group installation	Individual installation
Time for convencing	1 Session	4–5 Sessions
Self motivated	7 out of 8	No one
Age	16–50 years	4–40 years
Sex	Male-2, Female-6	Male-1, Female-4
Education	Till post-graduate	Till post-graduate

Conclusion: Group installation is superior to individual pump installation. Peer interaction helps in strengthening the learning process and smoothens insulin pump management.

19. Is CGM Essential for All Insulin Users to Prevent Hypoglycemia and GV—YES

Ritu Johari

ABSTRACT

Background: In recent decades, diabetes has seen tremendous advances in both therapeutic drugs as well as glucose monitoring technology. The question to address is what to choose when it comes to practical application – time-tested pre-existing glucometers to check glucose or newer continuous glucose monitoring (CGM) systems that display glucose 24×7 prick-free.

Objective: Validating use of CGM in Insulin users to avoid hypoglycemia.

Discussion: Glucose monitoring has always been a cornerstone for diabetes management. With advancement in technology within diabetes monitoring space, we now have newer metrics like the time in range (TIR) that take good glucose control to the next level for all types of diabetes. CGM is gaining increased attention in lieu of its 24×7 insights into real-time glucose trends and its ability to enable avoiding hypoglycemia and hyperglycemia in people living with diabetes.

Living with diabetes incurs huge expenses over one's pocket even when one is on oral anti-diabetic drugs (OADs). Insulin is usually reserved for later stages of the disease, when most OADs have been tried. Insulin therapy brings in weight gain and hypoglycemia as collateral damage. Hypoglycemia is another under-estimated entity that in different ways leads to raised morbidity and mortality in diabetes.

Hypoglycemia, more common with Insulin, has the potential to disrupt cerebral function. Statistics reveal 3.4 times higher mortality with hypoglycemia. Hypoglycemia, in many studies, is known to provoke cardiac events and death and thereby poorer patient outcomes. Besides, hypoglycemia may result in hospitalization from time-to-time causing both clinical as well as financial damage. Hence, avoiding hypoglycemia is a crucial step in diabetes management.

In an out-of-pocket, resource-crunched country, it is extremely critical to choose wisely between the popular inexpensive self-monitoring of blood glucose (SMBG) or the new CGM in Insulin users.

While SMBG may seem to be the easier choice, it is the CGM that comes across as the more economical option over a longer period of time through its benefits of better glucose control leading to lesser doctor visits, interventions and hospitalizations. Also, availability of pocket-friendly blinded CGM can also help diagnose hypoglycemia and potential hypoglycemia trends by doctors.

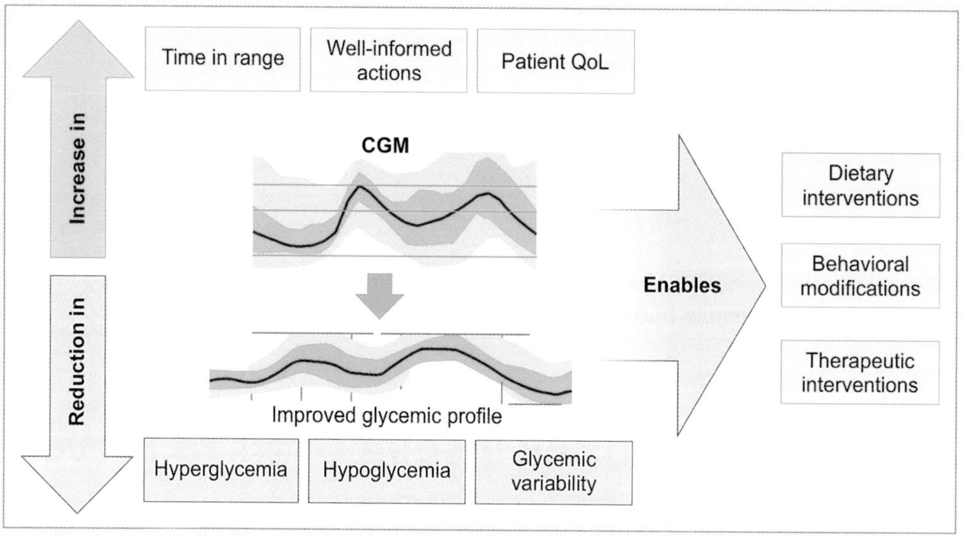

FIGURE 1: This figure illustrates the impact of CGM on multiple parameters like increasing the time spent in range (TIR), enabling well-informed actions by patient reducing hypoglycemia, hyperglycemia and glycemic variability, thereby improving patient's quality of Life (QoL). This tool provides opportunity to make dietary, behavioral as well as therapeutic interventions as and when required basis the displayed glucose journey. The AGP shown here is obtained using the FreeStyle Libre continuous glucose monitoring system by Abbott Diabetes care.

SMBG is a user-dependent tool and may miss many hyperglycemia and hypoglycemia events that are captured effortlessly with CGM. CGM also helps enable Insulin titrations that may or may not be accurate with SMBG. Many behavioral aspects such as defensive eating due to fear of hypoglycemia, under- or over-dosing Insulin based on food intake without knowing actual blood glucose level, may be avoided using CGM. CGM enables one visualize and learn the impact of various foods and activities on their glucose levels, thus understanding their diabetes much better and thus avoiding glucose fluctuations.

Conclusion: CGM, especially those that provide real-time insights, are a great tool to watch over glucose behaviors in Insulin users in any type of diabetes, both type I and type II, and help take well-informed decisions to enable avoiding hypoglycemia, hyperglycemia and even reduce glycemic variability. Hence, CGM is definitely an ESSENTIAL application for all Insulin users to prevent hypoglycemia.

20. Once weekly Insulin: Who, When and How

Parimal Swamy

ABSTRACT

Once-weekly insulin, an innovative approach to insulin therapy, holds promise for specific populations of patients with diabetes. Insulin Icodec and insulin Efsitora alfa are novel advancements in diabetes management, offering a once-weekly dosing regimen designed to improve adherence and glycemic control in patients with type 1 and type 2 diabetes. These innovations represent significant progress in simplifying insulin therapy, addressing common barriers such as the complexity of daily injections. Insulin Icodec has been approved for type 2 diabetes in several regions, with ongoing evaluations for type 1 diabetes. Insulin Efsitora alfa is currently under regulatory review.

The ONWARD clinical trials (ONWARD 1 to 6) investigated the efficacy, safety, and practical application of insulin Icodec. Similarly, the QUINT trials assessed insulin Efsitora alfa in diverse patient populations.

Who: Once-weekly insulin is particularly beneficial for adults with type 2 diabetes who struggle with adherence to daily insulin regimens, those with busy lifestyles, and individuals who experience treatment fatigue. It is also a potential option for newly diagnosed patients with poor glycemic control and those requiring basal insulin support. However, its use in type 1 diabetes remains limited due to unique insulin needs and variability in daily requirements.

When: This therapy is suitable for patients transitioning from oral hypoglycemic agents to insulin or those inadequately controlled on existing daily basal insulin regimens.

How: Once a week Insulins are administered subcutaneously once every 7 days, with a starting dose tailored to the patient's prior basal insulin regimen. Dose titration is typically based on weekly fasting blood glucose levels, ensuring a gradual and safe adjustment to achieve glycemic targets.

In conclusion, once-weekly insulin represents a significant advancement in diabetes care, offering convenience, improved adherence, and better quality of life for suitable patients. Its judicious use tailored to individual needs and clinical conditions, can optimize diabetes management while addressing long-standing challenges associated with daily insulin therapies. Further research is warranted to expand its indications and ensure equitable access to this promising innovation.

21. Insulin Pump for Everyone—YES

Anushree Mehta

ABSTRACT

The current standard of care for type 1 diabetes involves multiple daily insulin injections with frequent monitoring of blood glucose levels either with glucometers or with CGM devices. The current care requires the patient to be constantly involved in his diabetes management. No matter what one is doing, blood glucose and diabetes is always at the back of his mind. This leads to a significant burden on the PwD. Although Insulin pumps have been around for more than a decade, its adoption was limited due to the higher level of skills and training required with it. But, with the recent introduction of the Hybrid closed loop Insulin delivery systems or also called the Automated Insulin delivery systems this scenario has changed. It is a well documented fact that optimal HbA1c and target TIR can reduce risk of long term complications. Real-world studies for automated insulin delivery systems have shown improvement in HbA1c as well as TIR with minimal risk of hypoglycemia. Majority of the real world studies have reported a TIR of ≥ 70%.[1] Anybody living with or treating Type 1 Diabetes would realize how difficult it is to achieve consistent TIR of 70% with the current standard of care. Management of Type 1 Diabetes is incomplete without talking about psychological and quality of life outcomes. It has been reported that AID system is associated with reduced diabetes burden and improved well-being in people with diabetes.[2] Considering the above facts I would only ask 1 question—WHY NOT INSULIN PUMP FOR ALL?

REFERENCES

1. Considine EG, Sherr JL. Real-World Evidence of Automated Insulin Delivery System Use. Diabetes Technol Ther. 2024;26(S3):53-65.
2. Roos T, Hermanns N, Groß C, Kulzer B, Haak T, Ehrmann D. Effect of automated insulin delivery systems on person-reported outcomes in people with diabetes: a systematic review and meta-analysis. EClinicalMedicine. 2024;76:102852.

22. Active Play, Exercise and Sports with an AI Augmented Insulin Pump

Warren Lee

ABSTRACT

There are clear benefits of an active lifestyle and regular exercise in individuals without diabetes, but there are challenges in pursuing sports and exercise for people with type 1 diabetes, more so for those on insulin pumps. Exercise can result in better glycemic control but can cause euglycemia, hyperglycemia, even DKA or immediate and delayed hypoglycemia depending on the type and duration of exercise and the effects of underlying physical and mental stress, illness and effects of menstrual cycles. Will AI augmented pumps make things easier or harder? The principles of management for exercise for a patient on conventional and basal bolus insulin, conventional insulin pumps and AI augmented insulin pumps are compared. Conventional insulin pumps and MDI regimes may require behaviour modifications for safe exercise but a study on adherence to exercise guidelines suggests that guidelines requiring behaviour modification like meal and insulin dose changes are rarely followed. Prior hypoglycemia in the 24 hours pre exercise increases the risk of hypoglyemia associated with exercise, presumably because glycogen stocks in the body may not have been replenished after the previous episode, and reducing premeal insulin will be helpful for MDI and open loop pump regimes as will. Use of AID was associated with more spontaneity, less anxiety and less concerns about the guesswork needed to tweak insulin doses compared to open loop pumping. However, insulin sensitivity can drop significantly during exercise. The use of temporary target settings (for higher blood sugar) pre- and post-activity feeding would still be needed in some situations.

23. Experience Using AID in India and the Journey So Far

Jothydev Kesavadev

ABSTRACT

The journey of Automated Insulin Delivery (AID) systems in India spans nearly two decades, marked by continuous advancements and growing acceptance. This presentation outlines the evolution of AID systems, beginning with the introduction of insulin pump, MiniMed Medtronic Paradigm 722 in 2005 to the state-of-the-art AID MiniMed 780G in 2022. The AID systems have transformed diabetes care replacing conventional insulin pumps by integrating them with continuous glucose monitoring (CGM) and intelligent algorithms.

A case study highlights the real-world impact of AID systems: a female patient with fibrocalculous pancreatic diabetes (FCPD) transitioned through various technologies over 17 years. Significant improvements were achieved at each stage, including a reduction in average glucose levels, enhanced Time in Range (TIR) and improved QoL.

The advanced hybrid closed loop system (AHCL) available in India, MiniMed 780G, represents a milestone in automation, offering advanced features such as auto-basal-bolus adjustments, real-time glucose corrections, and predictive low-glucose management. These innovations address common challenges in diabetes care, including reducing glycemic variability, hypoglycemia and minimizing patient burden.

The adoption of AID systems in India initially faced barriers such as physician skepticism, high costs, and limited awareness. However, sustained efforts in education, training, and evidence-based practices have led to significant progress, with over 1,500 systems deployed across the country in just two years. Patient feedback emphasizes improved quality of life, reduced hypoglycemia, and greater ease of use.

This journey showcases India's evolving diabetes care landscape, emphasizing the pivotal role of AID systems in achieving better clinical outcomes and empowering people with diabetes.

Keywords: Automated Insulin Delivery, Insulin Pumps, Glycemic Control, Diabetes Technology, India

24. Recent Updates on Artificial Pancreas, Clinical Care and Next Steps

Ananda Basu

ABSTRACT

Automated Insulin Delivery (AID) – also known as Artificial Pancreas or Closed Loop Control – has come a long way since its inception > 50 years ago. Current AID systems are eminently portable, compact, safe, effective and user-friendly. In the US its use has been approved for patients with Type 1 Diabetes above the age of 2 years by the FDA. In multiple randomized controlled clinical trials, these systems have demonstrated improved glucose control with lowering of HbA1c while reducing the rates of hypoglycemia and hyperglycemia; improvements in hypoglycemia unawareness; significant mitigation of fear of hypoglycemia, disease burden and patient acceptability. Approved metrics derived from continuous glucose monitors (CGMs) have demonstrated increased percent time in range (TIR between 70–180 mg/dL) while lowering percent time below range (TBR < 70 mg/dL) and lowering percent time above range (TAR > 180 mg/dL). While such devices have not yet been approved in the inpatient arena, during pregnancy, following pancreatectomy and other pancreatogenous forms of diabetes (e.g., Cystic Fibrosis Related Diabetes), off-label use of AID systems in these states continue in the real world. Similar systems are also in use in Europe for patients with type 1 diabetes. Continuing research in AID systems include improvements in CGM technology (improved accuracy, multi-analyte capabilities); control algorithms (adaptive control, neural network, machine learning and AI incorporation); insulin pumps (tubeless, patch pumps) and dual/multi-hormone delivery (insulin + glucagon; insulin + amylin). It is hoped that in the next 5–10 years fully closed loop systems (i.e., without needing any patient input for meals, exercise) will be the norm.

25. Global Success of Automated Insulin Delivery as a Pathbreaking Innovation

Robert A Vigersky

ABSTRACT

There have been many breakthroughs over the last 100 years in the treatment of type 1 diabetes (T1D). Many of these have come in the last 10–20 years with the development and implementation of diabetes-specific technologies. Arguably, continuous glucose monitoring (CGM) and automated insulin delivery (AID) have been the most impactful in improving glycemic control. However, real-time CGM alone, i.e., in combination with a regimen of multiple daily injections, is insufficient for people with T1D to achieve the targets promulgated by the major international professional societies. The true value of real-time CGM is that it provides the input for algorithms that can automatically deliver (or suspend) insulin infusion up to every 5 minutes. Real-world results in tens of thousands of MiniMed™ 780G users demonstrate that the goal of >70% time-in-range (70–180 mg/dL; 3.9–10 mmol/L) is achieved in a substantial majority of people with T1D without an increase in time-below-range (<70 mg/dL; <3.9 mmol/L). These outcomes are remarkably similar across the globe regardless of race, ethnicity, diet, and culture suggesting that it has democratized the management of T1D.[1-3]

REFERENCES

1. Choudhary P, Arrieta A, van den Heuvel T, Castañeda J, Smaniotto V, Cohen O. Celebrating the Data from 100,000 Real-World Users of the MiniMed™ 780G System in Europe, Middle East, and Africa Collected Over 3 Years: From Data to Clinical Evidence. Diabetes Technol Ther. 2024;26(S3):32-7.
2. Shin J, et al. ATTD-Asia, Abstract 212. Diab Tech Ther. 2025, In Press.
3. Grassi B, Gómez AM, Calliari LE, Franco D, Raggio M, Riera F, et al. Real-world performance of the MiniMed 780G advanced hybrid closed loop system in Latin America: Substantial improvement in glycaemic control with each technology iteration of the MiniMed automated insulin delivery system. Diab Obes Metab. 2023;25:1688-97.

26. Why Automated Insulin Delivery is Standard of Care for the Treatment of Type 1 Diabetes

Robert A Vigersky

ABSTRACT

Real-time continuous glucose monitoring (CGM) when used with multiple daily insulin injections (MDI) provides a substantial improvement in glycemic outcomes in people with type 1 diabetes (T1D) over self-monitoring of blood glucose. However, multiple pivotal trial and real-world studies show that these glycemic outcomes are far from the goals [time-in-range (TIR) >70%] set by professional organizations. On the other hand, pivotal trials of automated insulin delivery (AID) systems and the real-world data from tens of thousands of people with T1D using commercially available AID systems demonstrate that they achieve TIR of 65–80% in children and adults and do so safely (time-below-range <4%). The differences in TIR between MDI+CGM versus AID systems range from 20 to 30%. Given the relationship of TIR to HbA1c,[1] this difference translates into a 1.5–2.4% difference in HbA1c. In addition, CGM-derived hyperglycemia metrics, i.e., time-above-range 180 mg/dL (10 mmol/L) are substantially higher than the consensus guideline recommendation of <25% in users of CGM+MDI, while most AID studies meet or are just above these goals. Given this overwhelming data, major national and international professional societies have promulgated increasingly more prescriptive guidelines stating that AID is the standard of care and the preferred method of treating all people T1D.[2] Furthermore, the National Health Service of the United Kingdom, recognizing the short- and long-term health implications and costs of inadequately controlled diabetes, has decided to make AID available at no cost to virtually all (~300,000) people with T1D.[3]

REFERENCES

1. Vigersky R and McMahon C. The Relationship of Hemoglobin A1C to Time-in-Range in Patients with Diabetes. Diab Technol Ther. 2019;21(2):81-5.
2. American Diabetes Association Professional Practice Committee. Erratum. 7. Diabetes Technology: Standards of Care in Diabetes-2025. Diabetes Care. 2025;48(Suppl. 1):S146-S166.
3. NICE recommends life changing technology is rolled out to people with type 1 diabetes. Available from [online] https://www.nice.org.uk/news/article/nice-recommends-life-changing-technology-is-rolled-out-to-people-with-type-1-diabetes. November 2023.

27. Immunotherapy for Type 1 Diabetes Prevention: Advances and Pitfalls

Stephen Greene

ABSTRACT

Type 1 diabetes (T1D) prevention strategies focus on delaying or halting disease onset by targeting its autoimmune nature.

Primary prevention aims to identify and intervene in genetically predisposed individuals before autoimmunity develops. Trials have explored dietary modifications, such as avoiding cow's milk or gluten, and antigen-specific therapies like oral insulin, but success has been limited due to challenges in identifying at-risk populations and ensuring safety.

Secondary prevention targets individuals with early-stage autoimmunity (presence of multiple autoantibodies). The FDA-approved drug teplizumab, an anti-CD3 monoclonal antibody, has shown promise in delaying T1D onset by modulating immune responses. Other approaches include using insulin or GAD65 antigens to induce immune tolerance, though to date the results are mixed.

Despite advancements, population-wide implementation is hindered by the complexity of genetic screening and the psychological burden on families. Future research should focus on refining risk stratification and improving the efficacy of interventions.

28. CGM Monitors be Recommended for All Patients with Diabetes Irrespective of Type—NO

Tejas Shah

ABSTRACT

Continuous glucose monitoring (CGM) devices have revolutionized diabetes management, offering real-time insights into blood sugar levels. However, mandating CGM for all types of diabetes is not a practical or equitable solution. First, not all individuals with diabetes require continuous monitoring. Type 2 diabetes, often managed through diet, exercise, and oral medications, typically does not necessitate the intensive tracking provided by CGMs. Fingerstick testing remains a cost-effective and sufficient option for many in this group.

Second, CGMs come with significant financial implications. These devices are expensive to purchase, maintain, and calibrate, creating a financial burden on healthcare systems and individuals, especially in low-income settings. Mandating their use for all diabetics would divert resources from other critical healthcare needs.

Furthermore, the utility of CGMs varies among patients. Not everyone benefits equally from the technology, particularly those with stable blood glucose levels or those who may struggle with the technical demands of CGM systems. Over-reliance on these devices could also lead to unnecessary anxiety or data overload for some users.

Lastly, promoting CGMs for all could inadvertently widen disparities in healthcare access, as underserved populations may face challenges in obtaining the technology despite its mandate. A one-size-fits-all approach ignores the individual needs and circumstances of people with diabetes.

While CGMs are transformative tools for managing certain cases of diabetes, their universal implementation for all types of diabetes is neither necessary nor efficient. Resources should instead be allocated based on individual needs, ensuring equitable and effective care.

29. An Analysis on Practical Tips for Recognizing and Addressing Insulin Inertia in Primary Care

Balaji Chidambaram

ABSTRACT

Aim: To analyze the Practical Tips for Recognizing and Addressing Insulin Inertia in Primary Care.

Objective: This study highlights practical tips and tools to recognize and address insulin inertia in primary care, aiming to enhance glycemic control and patient outcomes.

Methods:

- A comprehensive review of current diabetes management guidelines.
- Development of visual aids (algorithms, decision-making flowcharts) for insulin initiation.

Findings and Practical Tips:

- Early Recognition **Table 1:**
    - HbA1c levels persistently above target (>8% despite oral therapy).
    - High fasting blood glucose levels (>130 mg/dL).
    - Signs of beta-cell exhaustion (progressive hyperglycemia).

TABLE 1: Signs and triggers for insulin initiation.

Signs and triggers for insulin initiation	Description
Persistent hyperglycemia	Consistently high blood glucose levels despite oral medication or lifestyle changes
Fasting glucose > 130 mg/dL	Elevated blood sugar levels in the morning before eating
Postprandial glucose > 180 mg/dL	Elevated blood glucose after meals, often reflecting poor control of post-meal glucose spikes
HbA1c > 7.5–8%	HbA1c above the target range, indicating overall poor blood sugar control over time
Symptoms of severe hyperglycemia	Symptoms like excessive thirst, frequent urination, blurred vision, and fatigue
Progressive β-cell dysfunction	Worsening pancreatic insulin secretion due to progressive beta-cell dysfunction or insulin resistance
Failure of oral medications	When oral medications such as metformin, sulfonylureas, or DPP-4 inhibitors do not provide adequate blood glucose control

- Addressing Patient Concerns:
  - **Figure 1**: Common Patient Misconceptions and Rebuttals
  - Misconceptions (e.g., "Insulin means my diabetes is worsening"). Rebuttals (e.g., "Timely insulin use can prevent complications and improve quality of life").

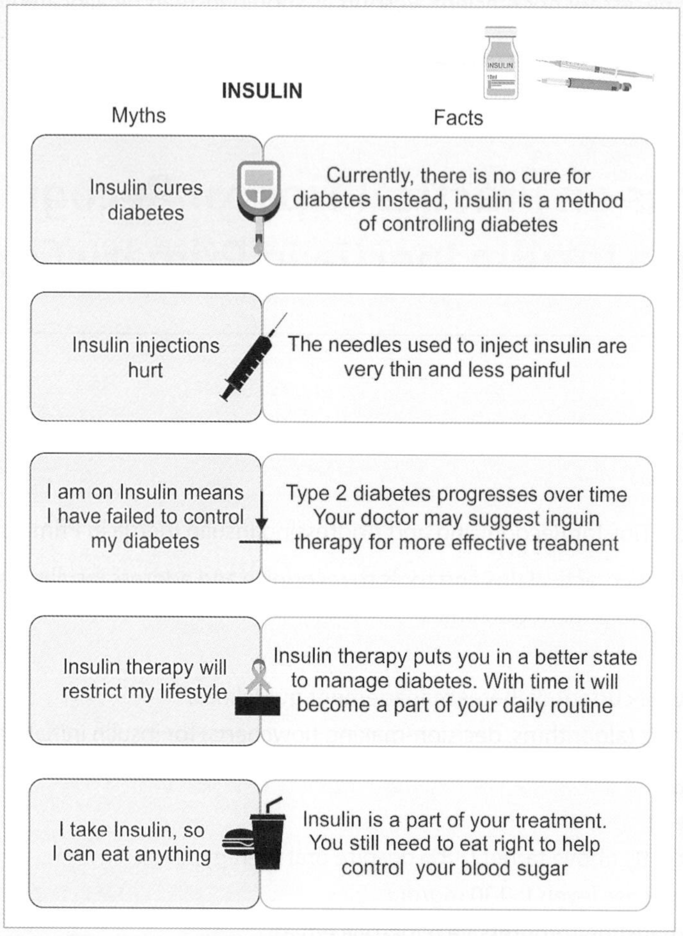

FIGURE 1: Common Patient Misconceptions and Rebuttals.

- Simplified Insulin Regimens:
  - **Flowchart 1**: Stepwise Approach to Insulin Titration in Primary Care.
- Overcoming Provider Barriers:
  - Encourage the use of digital tools for insulin dosing.
- Multidisciplinary Support:
  - Collaboration with diabetes educators and dietitians.
  - Integration of telemedicine

Conclusion: Addressing insulin inertia in primary care requires a combination of timely recognition, patient-centered communication and multidisciplinary support **(Fig. 2)**. Implementing these strategies can lead to improved glycemic outcomes and enhanced patient satisfaction.

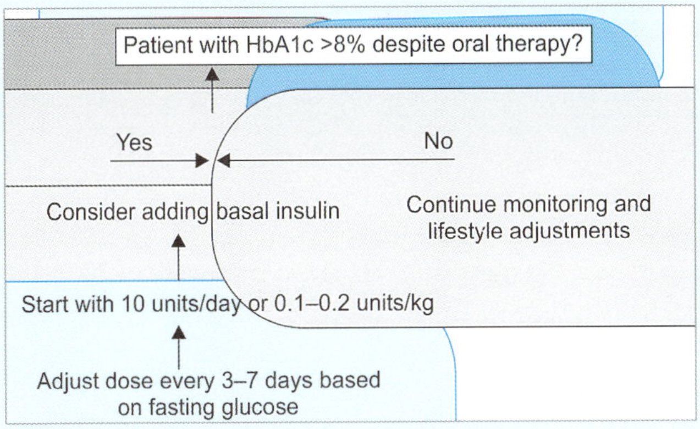

FLOWCHART 1: Decision tree for initiating and titrating insulin in primary care settings.

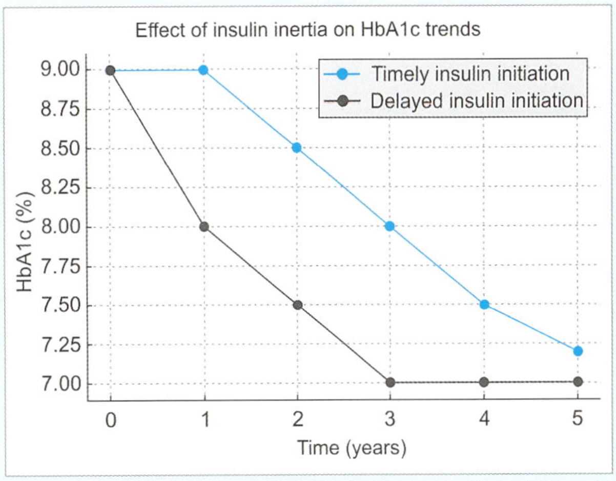

FIGURE 1: Graph depicting the Impact of insulin inertia on long-term A1c trends and complications

REFERENCES

1. American Diabetes Association. Standards of Medical Care in Diabetes—2025. Diabetes Care.
2. International Diabetes Federation (IDF). Global Guidelines for Diabetes Management.
3. Khunti K, et al. Insulin inertia and its impact on diabetes outcomes. Diabetes Ther. 2021.
4. Peyrot M, et al. Barriers to insulin initiation: Patient and provider perspectives. Diabetes Care. 2020.

30. Effect of Exercise Timing on Post Prandial Hyperglycemia

Ajoy Tewari

ABSTRACT

Exercise plays a crucial role in managing glucose levels and improving metabolic health. Postprandial exercise, particularly when initiated 10–30 minutes after a meal, significantly lowers glucose levels and enhances glycemic control. Both aerobic and resistance exercises are effective in blunting glucose spikes. Personalized exercise prescriptions, tailored to individual needs and preferences, enhance adherence and therapeutic outcomes. The timing of exercise is also critical, with post-meal exercise generally being more effective than pre-meal exercise. Short, frequent activity breaks and alternative exercises like stair climbing can be as effective as longer sessions for glucose management. Combining exercise with medications like metformin can further enhance glucose control and diabetes management. Future research should focus on optimizing exercise prescriptions, considering circadian rhythms, and exploring the synergistic effects of exercise and pharmacological treatments.

3
Section

Diagnostics and Biomarkers

31. Assessing the Predictive Value of Serum Creatinine and eGFR Values for CKD Status in T2DM

Ritu Johari, Pranjali Shah, Neeta Shah, Rukiya Shaikh

ABSTRACT

Background: Diabetes is a lifestyle disorder in which prevalence of chronic kidney disease is >25% and around 40% of people with DM develop chronic kidney disease during their lifetime. Within the general array of tests done for persons living with diabetes, routinely it is the creatinine levels that are considered for assessment of kidney function.

A search for the ideal endogenous marker of kidney function has been on since 1926. The Modification of Diet in Renal Disease (MDRD) equation for predicting GFR from serum creatinine concentration, developed by Levey AS, et al, 1999, has been recommended by researchers for routine use to predict GFR as more accurate estimates than those provided by creatinine clearance or the Cockcroft–Gault formula.

Aim: We aim to assess the predictive value of serum creatinine and eGFR values for CKD status in T2DM to ensure early intervention to prevent organ function from further deterioration.

Methods: We collected patient data from 4 different centres – mainly demographics like age, gender, duration of diabetes, body mass index, and laboratory values such as creatinine, blood urea nitrogen, eGFR, etc., and existing treatment regimens for T2DM patients irrespective of their kidney disease status.

Results: Off the 60 patients from 4 centres, gender was almost balanced in our subset. Age ranged from 41 to 85 years. Diabetes duration (1–30 years) and HbA1c, representative of glucose control (6.2% to 14%) were found somewhat associated with the eGFR. Approximately 38% patients had a normal creatinine level of less than 1. However, 92% had altered kidney function ranging from stage 2 to stage 4 CKD based on eGFR. Given the creatinine alone, actionable population was lesser than actual population, based on eGFR, qualifying for apt actions starting from strict glycaemic control and frequent monitoring of these parameters.

Conclusion: With the age of diagnosis reducing with time, and complications developing earlier in the journey of diabetes, one must look out for accurate indicators to diagnose CKD earlier in people living with diabetes. Erstwhile commonly used, serum creatinine is not truly indicative of the kidney function. eGFR is a single value that also takes age into consideration and provides a definitive picture of the kidney function enabling apt actions to prevent further deterioration of function.

Our study reinforces the migration to assess eGFR in addition to serum creatinine for understanding the exact kidney function in T2DM.

32. Ambulatory Glucose Profile (AGP): How can Clinicians get the Best Out of it?

Inge Van Boxalaer

ABSTRACT

Continuous Glucose Monitors (CGMs) have become indispensable in diabetes care, extending their utility beyond individuals with diabetes on insulin to those not on insulin, and even to people without diabetes, such as those with prediabetes or obesity. This growing adoption highlights the need for primary care physicians, nurses, and other healthcare providers to interpret CGM reports accurately and effectively.

This presentation introduces a simplified framework for interpreting Ambulatory Glucose Profile (AGP) reports, enabling healthcare providers to apply these insights systematically and teach them to others. Grounded in international guidelines, the framework begins with assessing data reliability, ensuring at least 14 days of CGM data with sensor usage exceeding 70%.

CGM reports provide actionable metrics such as:

- *Time in Range (TIR)*: The proportion of time glucose levels remain within 70–180 mg/dL (3.9–10 mmol/l), with a 5% TIR increase linked to clinical significant benefit.
- *Time Below Range (TBR)*: Ideally <4% of readings <70 mg/dL (3.9 mmol/), translated into minutes for better understanding.
- *Glycemic Variability (GV)*: A coefficient of variation ≤36% suggests stable glycemia.
- *Glucose Management Indicator (GMI)*: Reflecting estimated HbA1c from CGM data.

The AGP interpretation follows three systematic steps:

1. *Determine*: Review if TIR and TBR meet personalized goals, aiming for "More Green, Less Red" (MGLR).
2. *Where*: Identify problem areas in AGP curves, aiming for "Flat, Narrow, and In Range" (FNIR).
3. *To Act*: Confirm persistent patterns in daily graphs and adjust interventions accordingly.

Tailoring CGM alerts to minimize alarm fatigue is also emphasized. The presentation concludes with a quiz featuring real-life cases, equipping attendees with practical skills for CGM-guided diabetes care. By adopting this framework, healthcare providers can enhance patient outcomes through data-driven, personalized diabetes care.

AGP Report: Continuous glucose monitoring

Time in ranges goals for type 1 and type 2 diabetes

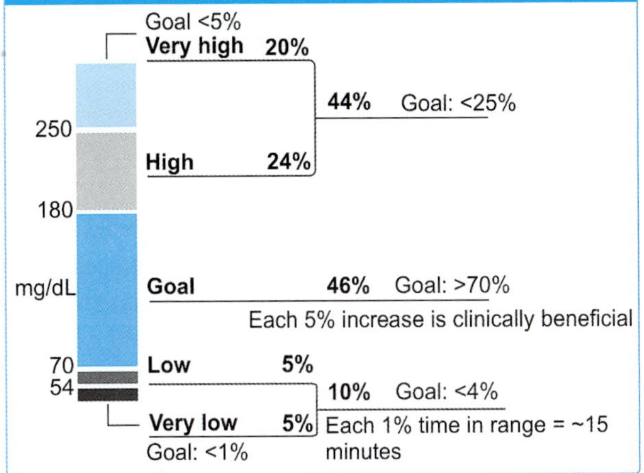

Test Patient DOB: Jan 1, 1970

14 Days: August 8–August 21, 2021

Time CGM Active: 100%

Glucose metrics

Average glucose............................**175 mg/dL**

Goal: <154 mg/dL

Glucose management Indicator (GMI)........**7.5%**

Goal: <7%

Glucose variability..................................**45.5%**

Defined as percent coefficient of variation
Goal: <36%

Ambulatory glucose profile (AGP)

AGP is a summary of glucose values from the report period, with median (50%) and other percentiles shown as if they occurred in a single day

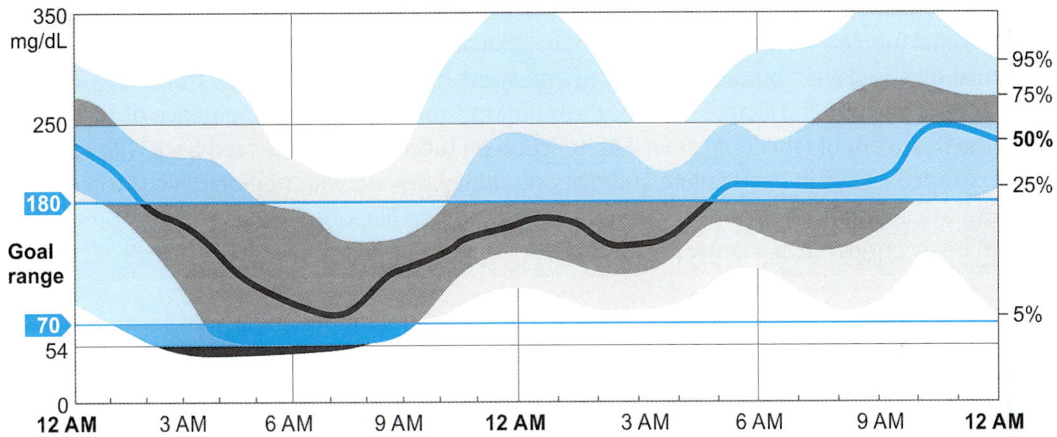

Daily glucose profiles

Each daily profile represents a midnight-to-midnight period.

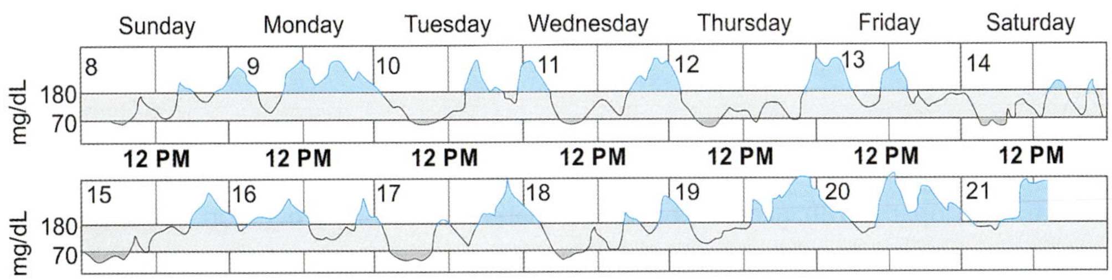

33. Renal Gluconeogenesis and Evolution of SGLT Receptor

Kamlakar Tripathi

ABSTRACT

The presence of SGLT receptors have been demonstrated in all metazoans like nematodes, molluscs, crabs, Gold fish as well as birds and mammals. During evolution the SGLT1 first appeared in gut epithelium to regulate the movement of glucose absorption which enters in eucaryotic cells via 2 different types of membrane associated carrier proteins, the Na^+-coupled glucose transporters (SGLT) and glucose transporter facilitators (GLUT). Three members of the SGLT family function as sugar transporters (SGLT1 and SGLT2) or sensors (SGLT3). As the animal adopted terrestrial life, the development renal tubular collecting duct increased the expression of SGLT2 to conserve sodium as well as water which increased to 90% in the proximal tubule and only 10% in gut. Subsequently GLUT emerged to carry glucose molecules to liver, muscles and adipocyte to convert in glycogen as well as substrate for fuel in different part of body and in cell for glycolysis and ATP generation. The human GLUT family consists of 14 members, of which 11 have been shown to catalyse sugar transport. The renal contribution to systemic gluconeogenesis is increasingly recognized. During the post-absorptive phase, the kidney accounts for ~40% of endogenous gluconeogenesis, occurring mainly in the kidney proximal tubule. The main substrate for renal gluconeogenesis is lactate and the process is regulated by insulin and cellular glucose levels, but also by acidosis and stress hormones. The kidney thus plays an important role in the maintenance of glucose and lactate homoeostasis during stress conditions. Emergence of SGLT2 inhibitors has revolutionized the treatment of type 2 DM as well as its action on tubulo glomerular feed back with sodium and water excretion has expanded its use in heart failure and diabetic kidney disease with non-diabetic chronic kidney disease. Newer indications are emerging and its use in non-diabetic condition like obesity, heart failure, proteinuria and CKD progression is to be reconsidered in a larger perspective.

34. Revolutionizing AI-powered Screening for Diabetic Retinopathy, AMD and Glaucoma

Bhavana Sosale, Srikanth Narayana, Usha Sharma, Sahana V Gowda, Aravind R Sosale

ABSTRACT

Background: Diabetic Retinopathy (DR), glaucoma and age related macular degeneration (AMD) coexist in patients with diabetes, causing vision loss if undetected. Comprehensive screening for multiple conditions can aid in early detection. The Medios artificial intelligence (AI) algorithm on the Remidio NM FOP (non-mydriatic fundus on phone camera) can screen for referable DR (RDR), AMD and glaucoma simultaneously. The potential of AI for integrated eye condition screening in diabetes care remains largely unexplored.

Aim: To screen for RDR, AMD and glaucoma using the Medios AI algorithm in patients with diabetes.

Methods: This was a cross sectional study of 1,591 patients with diabetes at Diacon Hospital in Bengaluru, India (September – November 2024). Mydriatic retinal images captured using the Remidio FOP camera were analyzed by the Medios AI, generating referral/no-referral reports for each condition.

Results: In this study 962 (60.4%) were men. RDR was present in 37%, referable AMD in 6.5% and disc suspect or referable glaucoma in 8.9%. Patients needing referral for at least 1 or 2 conditions was 50.3% and 2.5% respectively. Referable disease was higher in men.

Conclusion: One in three patients had RDR, and 1 in 2 needed referral for at least 1 condition. Comprehensive AI-powered screening in routine diabetes care can significantly improve early detection and management of multiple vision-threatening conditions. This study highlights the need for physicians to screen beyond DR while treating patients with diabetes. The Medios AI offers an opportunity to implement this approach effectively and transform eye health screening.

REFERENCE

1. Sosale B, Sosale A, Murthy H, et al. Simple, Mobile-based Artificial Intelligence Algorithm in the detection of Diabetic Retinopathy (SMART) Study. BMJ Open Diabetes Research and Care 2020;8:e000892.

35. Classification of the New Biomarkers

Kiran Shah

ABSTRACT

Glomerular biomarkers	Tubular biomarkers	Biomarkers of inflammation	Biomarkers of oxidative stress	Miscellaneous biomarkers
Albumin	Kidney Injury Molecule 1	Tumor necrosis factor- α	8oHdG, 8-oxo-7,8-dihydro-2-deoxyguanosine	VEGF, vascular endothelial growth factor
Transferrin	Neutrophil gelatinase-associated lipocain	Interluekin-1β		Nephrin
Laminin	Cystatin C	Interluekin-8 Interluekin-18		Podocalyxin
Ceruloplasmin	N-acetyl-β-D-glucosamine	Interferon gamma-induced protein 10		Retinol-binding protein
Immunoglobulin G	L-FABP liver-type fatty acid-binding protein	RANTES, regulated on activation, normal T cell expressed and secreted		AGEs, advanced glycation end products
Type IV collagen				
Glycosaminoglycans				
Fibronectin				

36. Non-invasive Glucose Monitoring Hype or Hope

Debashis Das

ABSTRACT

Glucose monitoring is an integral part of diabetes management and is key for medication adjustments, dietary guidance, tight glycemic control and complications prevention. Despite their reliability and accuracy, traditional invasive glucose monitoring methods present difficulties, such as discomfort, infection risk, and frequent calibration or blood sampling requirements. Over the past few decades, research has focused on developing non-invasive glucose monitoring (NIGM) technologies to address these issues. NIGM is a significant advancement in diabetes management, providing a more comfortable and convenient alternative to traditional invasive methods. This technology is intended to measure blood glucose levels without the need for finger pricks, thereby enhancing patient safety, compliance and quality of life. Various methods have been explored to achieve NIGM, including optical, electrochemical, electromechanical techniques. Each technique has its own set of challenges, particularly regarding accuracy, reliability, and sensitivity to physiological and environmental variables. Among all the techniques Photoplethysmography (PPG) and Near Infrared (NIR) Spectroscopy offer excellent acceptance and sensitivity and have been identified as the most promising resulting in having the most extensive application of machine learning. Despite these advancements, the pursuit of a universally acceptable non-invasive glucose monitoring device continues, driven by the need for improved accuracy and cost-benefit. The ongoing research and development activities are focusing on improving sensor technology, overcoming the environmental barriers, data processing algorithms, and device miniaturization. With wider application of artificial intelligence and machine learning, NIGM has the promise to transform diabetes care, making glucose monitoring more accessible, affordable and less burdensome for millions of people living with diabetes worldwide a greater hope to see few NIGM devices being available in the market soon.

37. New Biomarkers in Diabetic Kidney Disease: Are we there Yet?

Kiran Shah

ABSTRACT

Diabetic kidney disease (DKD) continues to be the leading cause of end-stage renal disease, and its global burden is increasing. DKD is linked to higher rates of cardiovascular disease and morbidity in all forms of diabetes. It is difficult to predict the course of DKD with albuminuria and eGFR, particularly in patients who are not proteinuric. While albuminuria is a sign of just glomerular damage, DKD's pathophysiology is complex and includes damage to all nephron components. To lessen the burden of DKD and ESRD, alternative and clinically meaningful early indicators are required, as evidenced by the limitations in urine albumin's diagnostic and prognostic significance. This will enable more focused and efficient diabetes treatment. Consequently, there is a paradigm shift toward new biomarkers that could aid in early DN risk prediction and potentially avert the development of end-stage kidney disease. These novel biomarkers have been broadly categorized as glomerular, tubular, inflammatory, oxidative stress, and miscellaneous biomarkers, which also include podocyte biomarkers, some of which are also categorized as tubular and glomerular biomarkers.[1] The bulk of them cannot yet be routinely used in clinical settings, despite their potential utility in the assessment of DN. Using EHR data and plasma biomarkers, a machine learned model called KidneyIntelX greatly enhanced the capacity to classify DKD patients as having low, intermediate, and high risk of progressive decrease in kidney function in order to improve outcomes. However, the emergence of new biomarkers is encouraging, and it is anticipated that in the future, physicians will have more access to a variety of tailored and efficient treatments for DKD patients.

REFERENCE

1. Uwaezuoke SN. The role of novel biomarkers in predicting diabetic nephropathy: a review. Int J Nephrol Renovasc Dis. 2017;10:221-31

38. Precision Medicine

Ranjit Unnikrishnan

ABSTRACT

The term "Precision Medicine" implies providing the right treatment to the right patient at the right time, based on sound scientific principles such as likely pathophysiology, genomics and differential response to treatment. The precision approach now has wide applications in all fields of medicine, and diabetes is no exception.

Precision medicine in prediabetes: The two common forms of prediabetes viz. impaired fasting glucose and impaired glucose tolerance, vary in prevalence, pathophysiology and response to intervention. Studies in western populations have identified distinct "clusters" of prediabetes that may differ in clinical outcomes, risk of complications and response to treatment.

Precision medicine in type 2 diabetes: Studies from European and Asian Indian populations (among others) have identified distinct subgroups of type 2 diabetes, based on clustering of easily measurable phenotypic variables. These clusters differ in ease of attaining glycemic control and risk of chronic complications. Studies are also underway to see whether they respond differentially to treatment modalities.

Precision medicine in type 1 diabetes: The role of precision medicine in type 1 diabetes is limited at present. Knowing the autoantibody status of individuals at risk of type 1 diabetes, or those in the early stages of disease, may help to identify them as candidates for preventive immunotherapy (e.g. Teplizumab).

Precision medicine in monogenic diabetes: Making an accurate molecular genetic diagnosis can inform treatment decisions in many cases of monogenic diabetes. Individuals with neonatal diabetes and some forms of maturity-onset diabetes of the young, may be able to stop insulin injections and go on oral sulfonylureas once a genetic diagnosis is made.

Conclusion: The precision approach has the potential to revolutionise diabetes care. However, more work needs to be done to define its role in the more common forms of diabetes. It should also be ensured that these investigations are available to all individuals with diabetes across the world so that health inequities are not worsened.

39. Early Diagnosis of Wolfram Syndrome Masquerading as Type 1 Diabetes with Complications

Kalpana Jog

ABSTRACT

Wolfram syndrome-1 (WFS1) is an autosomal recessive neurodegenerative, spectrum disorder characterised by early onset insulin dependent diabetes, optic atrophy, sensorineural deafness, diabetes insipidus (DI) and urodynamic dysfunction. These features evolve over time with an unpredictable order of emergence. Clinical diagnosis of WFS1 must be considered when a patient presents with any two or more of the above features. In spite of improved diagnostic methods including genetic testing this condition is still misdiagnosed as type 1 diabetes (T1DM). Early diagnosis helps to improve the quality of life.

Aims and Objectives: To develop a simple screening protocol which can be implemented by the medical caretaker to suspect WFS1 and differentiate from T1DM

Methods: Clinical and investigational profiles from T1DM record and mortality record were analysed for any clinical anomaly suggestive of WFS1.

We isolated 17 records out of which 13 were genetically confirmed WFS1, 1 deceased before testing, and 3 were misdiagnosed as T1DM with early complications, deceased at young age.

Based on our observations and analysis we developed a screening protocol which included testing for visual acuity (Snellen's chart), colour blindness (Ishihara's chart), hearing (ticking watch and phone apps) and olfaction (insulin smell). Fasting urine samples were tested for specific gravity by lab/reagent strip. In selective patients sonography for KUB was done.

Results: We have implemented screening protocol for each patient attending T1DM clinic since 2023. We suspected WFS1 in 5 patients. Investigated them further and confirmed genetically.

Conclusion: We can observe signs suggestive of multiple endocrine and neurological deficits early in the course of WFS1. Grossly impaired visual acuity, colour blindness, DI, deafness can appear way before noticeable optic atrophy. Our simple screening protocol ups the clinical vigilance to suspect WFS1 in the T1DM clinic enabling early diagnosis.

40. Sub-non Diabetic Hypoglycemia

Jaydip V Revale

ABSTRACT

Non-diabetic hypoglycemia (NDH) refers to low blood glucose levels in individuals without diabetes. NDH is relatively rare condition and can occur due to varies factors which can be intrinsic or extrinsic. Epidemiological studies have shown prevalence of NDH in admitted patients is 36 per 10,000 patients and common in older adults. NDH is children is mostly secondary to inborn errors of metabolism. NDH is characterized by imbalance between glucose production and utilization which is either insulin mediated or independent of insulin. Diagnosis of NDH requires detailed history, clinical examination and documentation of Whipple's triad. Extensive laboratory workup and imaging studies required to find root cause of hypoglycemia. Similar symptoms can be seen in many other conditions and should be ruled out by proper clinical evaluation. NDH is complex and potentially life-threatening condition which requires prompt recognition and treatment.

41. Managing Severe Insulin Resistance the Smart Way

Sambit Das, Sheenam Gupta

ABSTRACT

Insulin resistance (IR) is characterized by an impaired biological response to insulin, leading to subnormal glucose response. The causes of IR are multifaceted, involving genetic defects, secondary factors like stress and obesity, and specific hormonal or metabolic disorders. ACE identifies specific physiological abnormalities that increase IR risk, such as impaired glucose tolerance, dyslipidemia, and elevated blood pressure. Assessment of IR involves various indices and methods, with the hyperinsulinemic euglycemic clamp being the gold standard. Lifestyle interventions, including dietary modifications and physical activity, are crucial for managing IR. Dietary interventions include focus on calorie reduction, sodium reduction, and avoiding high glycemic load foods and consumption of non-starchy vegetables, minimizing added sugars and refined grains, choosing whole foods over highly processed foods. Choosing an exercise modality should be patient-specific and adopting a combination of both aerobic and resistance training seems to produce the greatest effect on insulin resistance. Aerobic exercise can directly augment insulin sensitivity, while resistance training boosts muscle mass that can positively affect glucose uptake Pharmacological interventions include drugs like Metformin and Thiazolidinediones, which improve insulin sensitivity and glucose control. Emerging therapeutic strategies target fat synthesis in the liver and skeletal muscle-specific agents to reduce IR. Suppression of lipid synthesis by use of agents targeting ACC1, ACC2, and DGAT2 which are in phase II clinical trials. Skeletal muscle-specific agents include uncoupling protein 3 activator and agents being developed to increase muscle quality, bezafibrate, which targets PPARs, is the subject of a phase II clinical trial on T2DM, and chiglitazar sodium, a PPAR pan-agonist, recently approved in China. Bariatric surgery has a role as it reduces adipose tissue volume and improves insulin sensitivity. Technology also plays by supporting weight loss and overall lifestyle improvements, by helping track calories, sleep hygiene, meal timing, and other personalized health data.

Treatment for insulin resistance should be based on multidisciplinary strategies that target physiological and metabolic impairments.

(IR: insulin resistance; ACE: American College of Endocrinology; ACC: acetyl-CoA carboxylase, DGAT: diacylglcyerol acyltransferase; PPAR: peroxisome proliferator-activated receptor)

42. How, What and Why of Abnormal Glucose Physiology

Rita Basu

ABSTRACT

The emergence of real time, accurate and continuous glucose sensing by continuous glucose monitors (CGMs) has revolutionized management of both type 1 and type 2 diabetes in the modern era. Prediabetes and type 2 diabetes, the prototypical chronic, progressive metabolic diseases are characterized by fasting and/or post prandial hyperglycemia to varying degrees. These dysglycemic patterns, occurring separately or together, are quickly recognizable with the CGM derived ambulatory glucose profiles (AGPs). However, it is important to understand the pathophysiological basis of dysglycemia that would help inform its rational management. Fasting hyperglycemia results from increased hepatic glucose production that in turn reflects abnormalities in glycogenolysis (in the early nocturnal period) and gluconeogenesis (in the late nocturnal period). These result from both inadequate insulin secretion as well as inappropriately elevated glucagon concentrations. On the other hand, post prandial hyperglycemia is related to reduced peripheral glucose uptake—due to peripheral insulin resistance; reduced hepatic glucose uptake—due to defects in hepatic glucokinase activity; and inadequate suppression of endogenous glucose production—due to inadequate suppression of post prandial glucagon concentrations and hepatic insulin resistance. It is important to note that systemic appearance of meal derived glucose is minimally, if at all, affected by either type 1 or type 2 diabetes unless gastric emptying is delayed (as in diabetic gastroparesis). Therefore, recognition of specific AGP patterns would inform targeted management strategies in the individual patient—especially with type 2 diabetes and prediabetes.

43. New Factors in the Control of Glucose

Hu Renming

ABSTRACT

There are many factors and pathways in the body that regulate blood sugar, such as diet, exercise, genetic diseases, mental states, and so on. Recent studies have proved that inflammation and inflammatory factors play an important role in regulating blood sugar. Products caused by metabolic disorders, such as lipopolysaccharide (LPS) and free fatty acids (FFA), often induce chronic low-grade inflammation, known as metabolic inflammation. Inappropriate food intake and decreased activity often lead to dysbiosis of the gut microbiota, with excessive gram-negative bacilli producing excessive LPS, which binds to toll-like receptors 4 on the surface of macrophages and inhibits microRNAs, thereby inducing polarization of the NF-κB system and producing inflammation. Polarized macrophages enter the intima of blood vessels to engulf cholesterol to form foam-like cells, which lead to AS; Polarized macrophages enter the invasion of pancreatic islets, the dedifferentiation of β cells leads to type 2 diabetes; Similarly, polarized macrophages are involved in the pathophysiological processes of fatty liver and obesity. Based on the high coexistence of T2DM, AS, NAFLD and overweight or obesity and the pathophysiological basis of chronic low-grade inflammation, Chinese diabetic workers proposed the concept of Metabolic Inflammatory Syndrome (MIS), suggesting that patients with 2 of the above 4 metabolic diseases can be diagnosed with MIS. Adiponectin was one of the most important soluble adipocytokines secreted mainly by white adipocyts had significant inhibitory effects on TNF-α–induced monocyte adhesion and pro-inflamatory cytokins expression in a dose depanded maner in vitro. In elderly inpatients (over 60 years old) hat lower serum adiponectin [OR = 22.937 (3.923–134.120)], higher fasting glucose levels ($p < 0.001$) were independently associated with MIS. The *TM4* gene Knockout mice present MIS cluster including T2DM, AS, Obese and fatty live.

Conclusion: T2DM is a component of metabolic inflammatory syndrome. Anti-inflammatory treatment is a potential targets for T2DM and MIS.

44. Pharmacogenomics in Diabetes

Shambo Samrat Samajdar

ABSTRACT

Type 2 diabetes (T2D) is a growing global health concern characterized by individual variability in drug response and tolerance, presenting significant challenges in effective management. Pharmacogenomics, the study of genetic influences on drug metabolism and efficacy, offers a promising pathway to personalized treatment strategies in T2D. This review explores the influence of genetic polymorphisms on the pharmacokinetics and pharmacodynamics of commonly used antidiabetic drugs, including metformin, sulfonylureas, thiazolidinediones, DPP-4 inhibitors, and SGLT2 inhibitors. Polymorphisms in genes encoding drug transporters (e.g., SLC22A1, SLC47A1), metabolizing enzymes (e.g., CYP2C9, CYP2C8), and drug targets (e.g., ABCC8, KCNJ11) significantly impact drug efficacy and safety, guiding therapeutic optimization.

Key insights highlight that preemptive genotyping can inform clinical decision-making, enabling tailored therapeutic regimens that enhance efficacy while minimizing adverse effects. For instance, genetic variants in SLC22A1 modulate metformin's glucose-lowering effects, while CYP2C9 polymorphisms influence sulfonylurea metabolism and hypoglycemia risk. Similarly, polymorphisms in WFS1 and PNPLA3 have been associated with differential responses to SGLT2 inhibitors, such as dapagliflozin. These findings underscore the necessity of integrating genetic testing into clinical practice, marking a shift from a "one-size-fits-all" approach to precision medicine in diabetes care.

Advancements in genomic technologies and reduced genotyping costs enhance the feasibility of implementing pharmacogenomics in routine practice, paving the way for a new era in T2D management that aligns with the principles of personalized medicine.

TABLE 1: Genetic variants and their impact on antidiabetic drug efficacy.

Gene	Protein	Polymorphism	Function	Impact on Drug Response	Drug Class
SLC22A1	OCT1	rs622342	Hepatic uptake of metformin	Affects therapeutic efficacy in certain ethnicities	Metformin
CYP2C9	Cytochrome P450 2C9	2, 3	Drug metabolism	Alters sulfonylurea metabolism and hypoglycemia risk	Sulfonylureas
ABCC8	SUR1	Ser1369Ala	KATP channel regulation	Modulates sulfonylurea effectiveness	Sulfonylureas
WFS1	Wolframin	rs10010131	Cellular homeostasis	Associated with weight loss in dapagliflozin users	SGLT2 Inhibitors
KCNJ11	Kir6.2	E23K	Pancreatic β-cell activity	Influences response to sulfonylureas	Sulfonylureas
PNPLA3	Adiponutrin	rs738409	Lipid metabolism	Affects liver fat reduction with dapagliflozin	SGLT2 Inhibitors
GLP1R	GLP-1 receptor	rs6923761	GLP-1 signaling	Impacts efficacy of liraglutide	GLP-1 Receptor Agonists

REFERENCE

1. Samajdar SS, Maheshwari A, Tiwari A, et al. Decoding the Genetic Blueprint: Advancing Personalized Medicine in Type 2 Diabetes through Pharmacogenomics. Clin Diabetol. 2024;13(6):386-396.

45. Genetics of Diabetes: Monogenic, Oligogenic or Polygenic

V Mohan

ABSTRACT

Diabetes has a large genetic component. However, its genetics varies depending on the type of diabetes. The common forms of diabetes like type 2 and type 1 diabetes are '*Polygenic*' with hundreds of loci which are associated with them but they are not casual.

'*Oligogenic*' diabetes refers to a condition when two or more genes are associated with some forms of diabetes. For example, Monogenic gene variants may be associated with type 2 diabetes also. Finally, the term '*Monogenic diabetes*' represents a group of disorders which are caused by mutation of a single gene. Monogenic diabetes is classified as those due to genes involved in insulin secretion and those due to genes involved in insulin resistance. The genes involved in insulin secretion include *neonatal diabetes (NDM)* defined as diabetes below 6 months of age and *maturity onset of diabetes of the young (MODY)*. MODY itself is of several different types, each with different clinical characteristics.

In addition, there are also other forms of monogenic diabetes like maternally inherited diabetes and deafness (MIDD) and genetic syndromes associated with diabetes. Most of the monogenic forms of diabetes are diagnosed based on genetic testing. The advantage of detecting monogenic forms of diabetes is that there could be therapeutic implications. For example, some individuals are wrongly diagnosed as having type 1 diabetes. If they found to have certain forms of monogenic diabetes like some forms of neonatal diabetes and MODY, they can be switched over to oral hypoglycemic agents (OHA). Each form of monogenic diabetes also has its own prognosis. Hence, it is important for the clinician to be aware of the various monogenic forms of diabetes and also when to order genetic testing for their diagnosis.

46. When and Why Screen for Thyroid and Celiac Disease

Warren Lee

ABSTRACT

Autoimmune thyroid diseases occur in 17–30% of patients with Type 1 diabetes (T1DM). Tests for Celiac Disease (CeD) are positive in 6–20% of people with TIDM. The prevalence of CeD is increased among first-degree relatives of children with T1D. CeD is frequently asymptomatic in children and young adults. CeD may present with gastrointestinal symptoms: diarrhea, bloat, nausea, abdominal pain and subclinical malabsorption, or extra intestinal features: Unexplained weight loss, iron deficiency anemia, decreased bone mineralization, aphthous stomatitis, poor growth and delayed puberty) or diabetes-related (unexplained hypoglycemia and unexplained hyperglycemia). CeD is an independent risk factor for retinopathy and nephropathy in T1DM patients. There diversity in clinical practices among physicians in diagnosing and managing CD in children with T1DM. In the ISPAD 2022 Guidelines screening for celiac disease is recommended during the initial year of diabetes diagnosis and at 2–5 years intervals, but in between formal screening points, when hypoglycemia is recurrent, it is important to rule out coexisting autoimmune disorders like subclinical hypothyroidism, celiac disease, and autoimmune adrenal insufficiency (Addison's disease). The gold standard for the diagnosis of CeD is the presence of vilous atrophy on intestinal biopsy (Marsh 3 grade and above), but endoscopic biopsies are often impractical or unaffordable. Revised recommendations for celiac disease (CD) screening include consideration of a serology-based diagnostic approach. The use of a single marker such has Tissue Transglutaminase 2 IgA (TTg IgA) is now being questioned and a 4 test panel including TTg IgG, Deamidated Gliadin Peptides (DGP) IgA, and DGP IgG is better for case finding. Some still use the Endomysial IgA test before considering biopsy, while the absence of HLA DQ2 and DQ8 alleles should no longer be used to exclude the possibility of Celiac Disease.

47. Algorithm for Assessment of MASLD in Patient with Diabetes

Wahid Khan

ABSTRACT

Overview: MASLD and T2DM are prevalent metabolic disorders; They often coexist and exacerbate each other.

Key mechanisms: Insulin resistance, inflammation, lipotoxicity.

Prevalence and Impact: T2DM: 800 million individuals in 2024; Expected to rise to 1.23 billion by 2050.

MASLD: Patients with T2DM have a higher prevalence of NAFLD (ranging from 30 to 75%) and a higher risk of developing NASH with fibrosis.

Pathophysiological Pathways

- *Insulin Resistance*: Disrupted glucose metabolism; Chronic hyperinsulinemia.
- *Lipotoxicity*: Accumulation of harmful lipid by-products.
- *Adipocyte Dysfunction*: Increased cytokine production.
- *Microbiota Dysbiosis*: Role of Microbiota—changes in gut flora contribute to MASLD and T2DM; Increased intestinal permeability and dysbiosis.
- *Bile Acid Metabolic Pathways*: Bile Acid Receptors—FXR and TGR5; Regulation of glucose and lipid metabolism.
- *Genetic Factors*: Over 400 genomic regions linked to T2DM; Key genes: PNPLA3, HSD17B13, MBOAT, TM6SF2.

Clinical Implications:

- *Surveillance*: Regular screening for T2DM in MASLD patients; Importance of glycemic control.
- *Microvascular complications*: Increased risk of CKD and diabetic neuropathy.
- *Cardiovascular disease*: Leading cause of death in T2DM and MASLD.

Diagnosis and Staging:

- *MASLD diagnosis*: Criteria: liver steatosis, cardiometabolic risk factors, exclusion of other causes; Preferred methods: ultrasound, MRI-PDFF, CAP.
- *Fibrosis Assessment*: Non-invasive tests: FIB-4, elastography.

Summary of Diagnosis and Assessment of MAFLD/NAFLD

- *Diagnosis*: NAFLD is diagnosed with ≥5% hepatic steatosis, primarily via conventional ultrasonography.
- *Fibrosis assessment*: Using blood tests or liver stiffness measurements.
- *Liver stiffness*: Transient elastography (e.g., FibroScan®) assesses liver stiffness; MRI-PDFF is the gold standard for quantifying hepatic steatosis.
- *Advanced disease assessment*: Non-invasive tests like FIB-4 and ELF test estimate advanced fibrosis.
- *Endoscopic screening*: Patients with LSM >15 kPa and platelet count <150,000 should be screened for varices.

Diagnosis: Protocol for evaluation of NAFLD

- Patients could be asymptomatic or complain of complain of unexplained fatigue and RUQ discomfort. incidental discovery of steatosis also indicates comprehensive evaluation
  - Family and personal history of NAFLD-associated diseases
  - Exclusion of secondary causes of steatosis

Level	Variable
Initial evaluation	• Alcohol intake: <20 g/day (woman), <30 g/day (men) • Personal and family history of diabetes, hypertension and CVD • BMI, waist circumference, change in body weight • Hepatitis B/hepatitis C virus infection • History of steatosis-associated drugs • Liver enzymes (ALT, AST, GGT) • Fasting blood glucose, HbA1c, OGTT, (fasting insulin [HOMA-IR]) • Complete blood count • Serum total and HDL cholesterol, triacylglycerol, uric acid • Ultrasonography (if suspected for raised liver enzymes)
Extended evaluation	• Ferritin and transferrin saturation • Tests for coeliac and thyroid diseases, polycystic ovary syndrome • Tests for rare liver diseases (wilson, autoimmune disease, AATD)

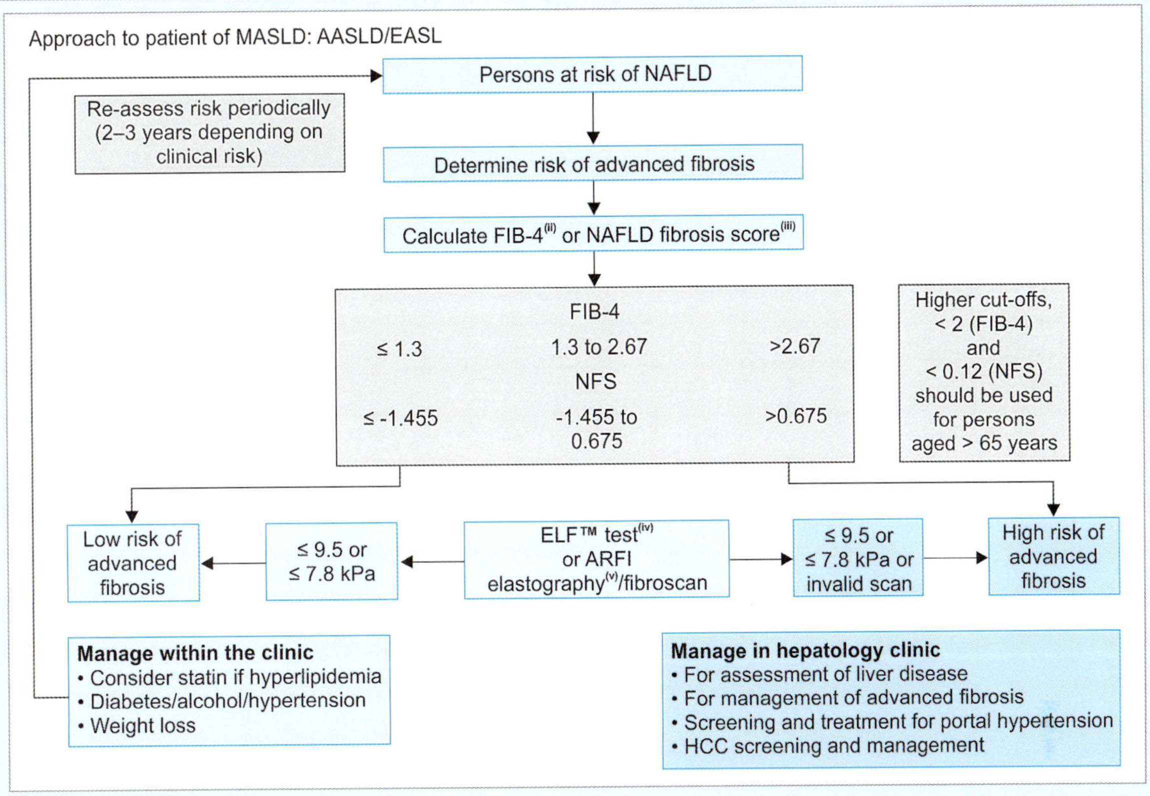

FLOWCHART 1: Approach to patient of MASLD: AASLD/EASL.

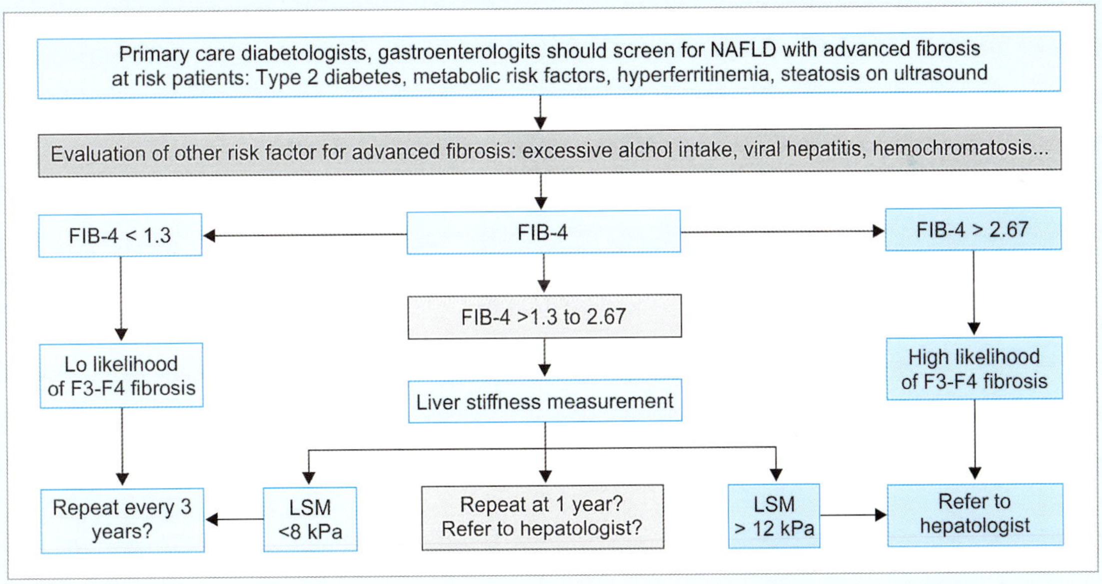

FLOWCHART 2: Clinical care pathway for the risk stratification and management of patients with NAFLD.

4
Section

Technological Advances in Diabetes Care

48. Debate: Fixed Dose Combination (FDCs) is Boon for Primary Care Physician (Favor)

Deepak Kumar Das

ABSTRACT

Definition: FDCs are medications that contain two or more active pharmaceutical ingredients in a single dosage form.

Examples: Anti-hypertensives: Telmisartan + Hydrochlorothiazide, Anti-diabetics: Metformin + Sitagliptin, Antibiotics: Amoxicillin + Clavulanic Acid

Purpose: To enhance therapeutic efficacy and patient compliance

Relevance in Primary Care:

- Simplified prescribing
- Simplify treatment regimens for chronic diseases.
- Improve medication adherence by reducing pill burden.
- Cost-effective for patients due to single packaging.
- Reduction in hospitalizations due to better disease control and also enhanced patient satisfaction.
- Broad-spectrum solutions for infectious diseases.

Benefits of FDCs:

- *Improved Adherence*:
  - Simplifies complex regimens.
  - Enhances patient convenience.
- *Enhanced Efficacy*:
  - Synergistic effects of combined agents.
- *Reduced Resistance Risk*:
  - Combination therapy lowers the chances of microbial resistance.
- *Lower Healthcare Costs*:
  - Decreased need for separate medications and frequent monitoring.
- Measures to Promote Rational FDCs

  A multistep and multistakeholder approach is necessary to improve the rationality of prescribing FDCs. Necessary to ensure good pharmacovigilance, a rationale to develop FDCs, good prescribing and pharmacy practices, active enforcement by regulators. Continuing medical education of medical and pharmacy students with regard to drug information

Conclusion:

- FDCs as a pragmatic solution for primary care physicians to enhance patient care.
- They improve compliance, outcomes and cost-efficiency.
- Awareness and regulation are key to addressing associated risks.

49. Do Devices Help a Person with Diabetes?

Aravinda J

ABSTRACT

Background: Diabetes is a major global health crisis, with innovative technologies offering promise for enhanced management.[1]

Objective: The study aims to investigate the efficacy of diabetes management devices, CGM and insulin pumps, in improving glycemic control and quality of life for individuals with diabetes.

Method: Relevant articles published between 2000 and 2020 were retrieved from electronic databases (Google Scholar and PubMed) using "devices AND type 2 diabetes mellitus" as keywords.

Results: Real-time Continuous Glucose Monitoring (rtCGM) improve outcomes for individuals at high risk of hypoglycemia, those with significant glycemic variability, and specific populations such as pediatric and elderly patients. In contrast, intermittently scanned continuous glucose monitoring (isCGM) benefited patients struggling with self-monitoring, facilitating informed treatment decisions.[2] Meta-analysis results indicate that rtCGM increases time-in-range (TIR) by 7%. No significant difference in HbA1c levels was found between rtCGM and isCGM. It was reported that rtCGM provides superior glycemic benefits over isCGM for Type 1 Diabetes patients, underscoring the need for improved access and affordability.[3] A Study finding reveals that using insulin pumps to maintain near-normal blood glucose levels significantly reduces the risk of eye, kidney, and nerve complications, and insulin pump users were found to have a lower mean A1c than MDI users.[4]

Conclusion: CGM sensors and insulin pumps are transforming diabetes management, improving therapy safety and effectiveness, reducing hypoglycemia, and decreasing glycemic variability. Despite benefits, adoption is hindered by insurance coverage, cost, provider bias, and technology attitudes, highlighting the need to address disparities and barriers.

Keywords: Glycemic control, continuous glucose monitoring, insulin pump

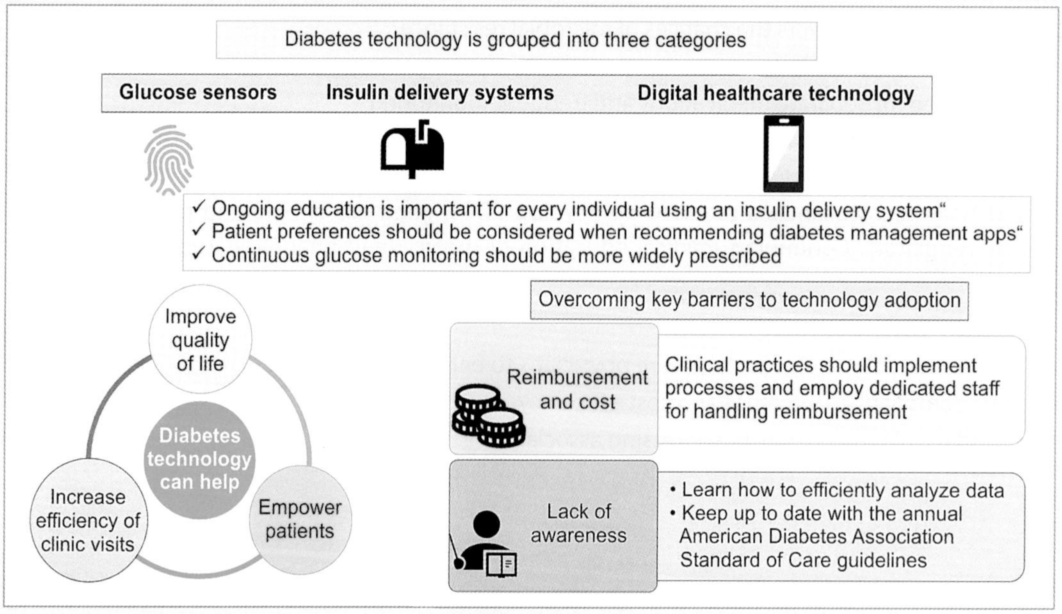

REFERENCES

1. Huang X, Yao C, Huang S, et al. Technological Advances of Wearable Device for Continuous Monitoring of In Vivo Glucose. ACS sensors. 2024;9(3):1065-88.
2. Chamberlain JJ, Doyle-Delgado K, Peterson L, et al. Diabetes Technology: Review of the 2019 American Diabetes Association Standards of Medical Care in Diabetes. Annals of internal medicine. 2019;171(6):415-20.
3. Zhou Y, Sardana D, Kuroko S, et al. Comparing the glycaemic outcomes between real-time continuous glucose monitoring (rt-CGM) and intermittently scanned continuous glucose monitoring (isCGM) among adults and children with type 1 diabetes: A systematic review and meta-analysis of randomized controlled trials. Diabet Med. 2024;41(3):e15280.
4. Gandhi K, et al. Clinical diabetes: a publication of the American Diabetes Association, 42(1), 56–64.

50. Continuous Glucose Monitoring in Diabetes Management: Do they Really Help?

Vivien Lim

ABSTRACT

Continuous Glucose Monitoring (CGM) has revolutionised clinical management of diabetes in many ways, not just conventionally in terms of HbA1c improvements, but also ease of monitoring and ability to educate patients on presence of carbohydrates in different foodstuff. These devices measure glucose levels in the interstitial fluid and provide a measurement of glucose level 24 hours without fail over a varied time period depending on the CGM device.

The talk aims to give a brief overview to familiarise the audience with usage of the device and interpretation of the data. There will be case studies that will illustrate the various advantages that use of CGM confers to the management of diabetes. Amongst them are the following:

- Improvement of HbA1c – via various mechanisms
- Familiarity with carbohydrates and hence ability to moderate it and as a consequence having a salubrious effect on weight
- Analysis of glucose trends to enable better matching of insulin with food in those who are on bolus regimens
- Aid in optimising management for the patient be it hyperglycemia and selection of drugs or hypoglycemia

51. POCT: The Right Tool to Meet the Urgent Needs of the Diabetes Clinic

Bijay Patni

ABSTRACT

Point-of-care testing (POCT) is increasingly essential in diabetes management, providing rapid diagnostic capabilities that enhance patient care and treatment outcomes. Various POCT modalities facilitate immediate assessments critical for effective diabetes management. Key tests include HbA1c testing using devices like HemoCue and Roche's Cobas b

101, which enable timely treatment decisions based on long-term glucose control. Blood glucose monitoring through glucometers allows quick responses to hyperglycemic or hypoglycemic events. Additionally, point-of-care lipid profile tests provide immediate results for cholesterol levels, aiding in cardiovascular risk management among diabetic patients. Urine analysis, including the Urine Albumin-to-Creatinine Ratio (UACR) test, is vital for assessing kidney health, while continuous glucose monitoring (CGM) systems are gaining traction for their ability to provide real-time glucose readings. The advantages of POCT include improved timeliness of results, enhanced patient engagement, and streamlined clinical workflows. However, challenges such as standardization of testing procedures, the need for provider training, cost considerations, and quality assurance must be addressed to maximize the benefits of POCT in diabetes care. A study by Saboo et al. (2019) emphasizes the importance of implementing structured POCT protocols in clinics to optimize diabetes management and improve patient outcomes. Integrating various POCTs in diabetes clinics significantly enhances patient management by providing rapid and accurate diagnostic information. As the prevalence of diabetes continues to rise globally, the role of POCT in facilitating timely diagnosis and personalized management becomes increasingly critical.

REFERENCES

1. Lenters-Westra, E. (2023) HbA1c Point of Care Testing: Is It Good Enough for Clinical Practice? [online]. Available at: https://diagnostics.roche.com/global/en/article-listing/hba1c-point-of-care-testing-for-clinical-practice.html (Accessed: 14 January 2025).
2. Ghosh, A., et al. (2023) Point-of-care diagnostics for diabetes: Progress and prospects [online]. Available at: https://www.researchgate.net/publication/373398491_Point-of-care_diagnostics_for_diabetes_Progress_and_prospects/download (Accessed: 14 January 2025).
3. Saboo B, et al. (2019) Recommendations for in-clinic PoCT for diabetes management Diabetes & Metabolic Syndrome: Clinical Research & Reviews, 13(1), pp. 5-7.

52. Moving from Beta Cells to Brain to Treat Diabesity

Vinod Mittal

ABSTRACT

India has one of the highest numbers of people with diabetes in the world. As per ICMR-INDIAB study there are nearly 101 million adults in India have diabetes, with numbers expected to rise exponentially by 2045. Current treatment focuses on increasing insulin secretion by pancreatic β-cells, improving insulin action on liver, fat, muscle and favoring renal glucose elimination.

Neuronal circuits in the brain, in particular in the hypothalamus and brainstem, can exert strong control on glucose homeostasis. When activated, these neuronal circuits can regulate, by controlling autonomic nervous system activity, the secretion of insulin and glucagon by pancreatic endocrine cells as well as glucose metabolic pathways in liver, fat, and muscle.

New therapies can act on different mechanisms like hypothalamic signaling systems (regulation of insulin sensitivity, glucose and lipid metabolism, feeding behavior, control of functions of the nervous, endocrine and cardiovascular systems), insulin/IGF-1 signaling (intranasal route of insulin delivery), Inhibition of PTP1B (insulin resistance and metabolic disorders), Dopamine signaling system (cognition, emotions, feeding behavior), Serotonin signaling system, melanocortin signaling system (regulation of blood glucose, insulin sensitivity, feeding behavior and lipid metabolism). GLP-1 RAs also act on brain to achieve early satiety and decrease appetite, having tremendous effect on weight reduction in addition to control of glycemia.

Gut-brain-microbiota axis also has a robust influence on weight and hyperglycemia through their relationship with the host metabolism and implications in several pathways.

Conclusion: In summary, the idea of "moving from Beta Cells to Brain" represents an integrated approach to treating diabesity by addressing both the pancreas and the brain, key regulators of glucose metabolism and body weight. This multifaceted strategy holds promise for more effective and comprehensive therapies.

53. Innovations in Footwear Technology to Prevent Diabetic Foot Ulcers

Sanket Pendsey

ABSTRACT

Footwear is not only preventive but also helps in treating a patient with diabetic foot ulcer (DFU). However, inappropriate footwear can also be the cause of DFU. Hence, it is essential to prescribe every patient especially with at risk feet with a correct footwear. Despite better understanding of the role of footwear in preventive foot care, in clinical practice we often come across patients using custom moulded footwear which fails to either offload or ensure pressure redistribution. This gap can be filled by using technology.

Just like we have smart phones, smart city, etc., we now have smart shoes too. Amongst the many factors that help in preventing ulcer recurrence, monitoring foot skin temperature and plantar pressures are most vital aspects. Smart shoes can monitor skin temperature as well as give valuable information about plantar pressures which can help to design bespoke insoles.[1] In addition, Smart footwear can also help in gait analysis, sweat measurement, information about rotational and tilting movements of the foot while walking.

Use of 3D scanning and printing technology can be helpful in designing more accurate customised footwear especially for those with deformity. Newer insole materials such as PORON, EVA or plastozote may be more effective in plantar pressure redistribution during walking as compared to barefoot walking and normal footwear.[2]

A compounding factor in DFU is development of infection which can be fungal or polymicrobial. Footwear coated with antifungal and antimicrobial properties such as silver ions have shown to reduce incidence of diabetic foot infections.[3]

Innovative footwear assisted with newer technology is definitely transforming the care of people with a DFU. Making it evidence based, accessible and affordable is the key to ensure that such footwear reaches maximum number of people with diabetes.

REFERENCES

1. Rukmini PG, Hegde RB, Basavarajappa BK, et al. Recent Innovations in Footwear and the Roleof Smart Footwear in Healthcare—A Survey. Sensors 2024;24:4301.
2. Shi QQ, Li PL, Yick KL, et al. Effects of contoured insoles with different materials on plantar pressure offloading in diabetic elderly during gait. Sci Rep. 2022;12:15395.
3. Marques SM, Carvalho I, Leite TR, et al. Antimicrobial TiN-Ag Coatings in Leather Insole for Diabetic Foot. Materials 2022;15:2009.

54. Metabolic Medicine 2030: What the Future will Bring

Ananda Basu

ABSTRACT

Management of chronic metabolic diseases of which Type 2 diabetes is the putative "poster child" has come a long way in the past decade with emergence of novel therapeutic strategies. These include, but are not limited to modulators of incretin axis and related hormones (dual agonists), glycosuric agents (SGLT2 inhibitors) and very long acting insulin analogs (Insulin Icodec). Current research and development predicted in the next decade involves dual and triple agonists (GLP-1 + GIP + GCGR agonists), smart insulins (glucose dependent insulin release), glucose sensitive insulin release using nano-technology, glucagon receptor agonists/antagonists, GPCR40 agonists, ghrelin analogues, glucokinase activators, GLUT4 transporter stimulators and PT1B antisense oligonucleotide inhibitors amongst others. Another rapidly evolving concept is the emergence of precision medicine for diabetes management that will replace the current "shotgun" approach with targeting specific phenotypes of Type 2 diabetes based on body habitus and markers of beta cell function and autoimmunity. These sub-phenotypes of Type 2 diabetes have been well documented in the Scandinavian and US populations that could lend themselves to initial and informed management with insulin sensitizers versus secretagogues versus incretin-based therapeutics. Furthermore, a better understanding of pathogenesis of Metabolic Dysfunction-Associated Steatohepatitis (MASH) will lead to specific strategies in its co-management along with co-existing type 2 diabetes. The role of epigenetics in the development of these metabolic disorders could also lead to innovative approaches such that in the next 20–25 years current therapies could become obsolete and consigned to the realm of historical facts!

55. Use of AI in Day to Day Clinical Practice? Is It Really Working?—YES

Hamid Ashraf

ABSTRACT

Global healthcare systems have significant challenges in achieving the quadruple aim: strengthening population health, improving patient care experiences, increasing caregiver satisfaction, and reducing healthcare costs.

Ageing populations, growing chronic illness rates, and rising healthcare expenditures are forcing governments, payers, and regulators to innovate and reform healthcare delivery systems.

AI may help healthcare systems achieve their 'quadruple purpose' by democratising and standardising networked, AI-enhanced care, precision diagnostics, treatments, and drugs. AI research in healthcare is advancing quickly, showing industry-wide applications.

AI is being integrated into diabetes treatment, although many clinics are still researching or deploying it. Diagnostics and risk assessment are significant AI uses. AI is increasingly diagnosing diabetic retinopathy. AI/ML image processing is becoming increasingly common and accurate. This technique is advantageous in our resource-constrained country.

Recent research from our institute shows that corneal and conjunctival images may identify diabetes mellitus with 95% accuracy. We recently showed AI/ML can accurately predict diabetic nephropathy using clinical data.

AI-based insulin pumps significantly benefiting patients reliant on insulin for hyperglycemia control. AI holds significant promise for delivering precise therapy to individuals with diabetes mellitus. Artificial intelligence is helpful in analysing continuous glucose monitoring (CGM) records of patients, enabling precise predictions of hypoglycemia. AI-based chatbots are increasingly often used in our clinics to provide instruction on nutrition, insulin administration, storage, and hypoglycemia. AI-enabled applications provide the remote transmission of CGM data, blood glucose measurements, and other health information from patients to their healthcare professionals. AI systems evaluate this data and provide tailored feedback, enhancing remote management.

AI helps with administrative, scientific, and therapeutic goals. AI helps optimise clinical trials and pharmaceutical development by managing and comprehending large amounts of data.

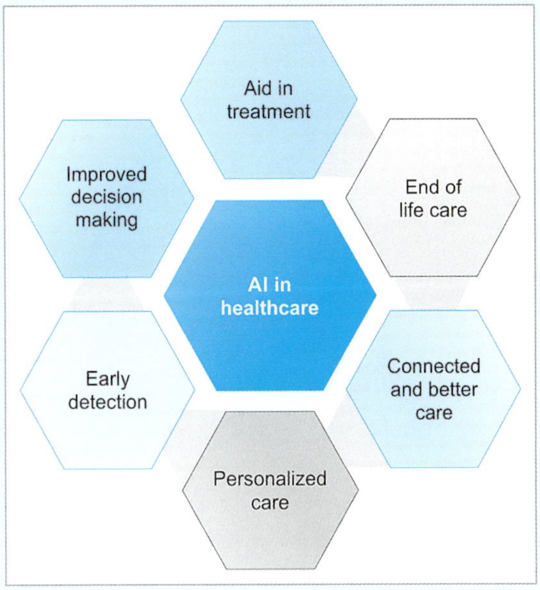

FIGURE 1: Use of AI in diabetes management.

56. Advanced Carbohydrate Counting, on 14th February 2025

Smita Shah

ABSTRACT

Carbohydrate counting is a fundamental aspect of diabetes management. This presentation explores the application of advanced carbohydrate counting as a personalized strategy to optimize glycemic control and enhance patient care. By integrating the impact of macronutrients, Glycemic Index (GI), and Glycemic Load (GL) into meal planning, and incorporating insulin sensitivity factor (ISF) calculations, this approach enables tailored insulin-to-carbohydrate ratios and precise blood glucose adjustments. This presentation aims to equip healthcare professionals with practical insights into implementing advanced carbohydrate counting in clinical practice. By adopting this refined approach, patients can achieve tighter glycemic control, reduce the risk of complications, and enhance their overall quality of life.

5
Section

Clinical Approaches and Guidelines

57. How do we Care our Elderly with Diabetes?

Vinod Kumar

ABSTRACT

Lifestyle and drug prescription apart, two more prescriptions, functional prescription and social prescription are required for better caring for elderly diabetics who are often more prone to functional decline compared to non-diabetic elderly.

Functional prescription aims to prevent age-related decline in various functions such as cognition, mobility, vitality (nutrition), vision, hearing and psychology-all collectively termed as intrinsic capacity (IC) by WHO. Simple training is required to screen these functions as evident from WHO's quick 10-minute tool (https://youtu.be/92qX9IVWsrl?si=iYMFdY4NTaqRz1ge)[1] developed by its Integrated Care for Older People (ICOPE) program for health workers, doctors to use for older persons. Used for older diabetics also.[2-4] In case any of the above 6 domains of IC is impaired, further preventive measure in the form of cognitive stimulation, exercises, diet, eye care, ear care and psychological support respectively can be provided through proper referrals or/and an in-depth Comprehensive Geriatric Assessment (CGA) by geriatrician to help detect and manage geriatric syndromes like dementia, frailty, falls, depression etc. Both ICOPE Screening tool for IC and CGA help stratify functional health of older diabetics to improve diabetes care through individualizing the management, determining treatment goals, and assessing and strengthening diabetes self-managing abilities. This also supports a person-centred holistic approach as a useful addition to well-established comprehensive diabetes evaluation (CDE).[5]

Social prescription by doctor to connect patient with non-clinical activities at voluntary and community sectors lead to improved health including better glycaemic control.[6] Examples are music, new reading, new language, gardening, fun with games, befriending children, exploring the internet, knitting, cooking, cleaning the environment, tutoring, spirituality, volunteering etc. This needs to be formalized and integrated in diabetes care.[7]

REFERENCES

1. WHO 2019(WHO/FWC/ALC/19.1
2. 10.26502/acmcr.96550574
3. https://ssrn.com/abstract=4449100
4. https://doi.org/10.1016/j.archger.2024.105687
5. https://doi.org/10.1002/9781118954621.ch5
6. https://doi.org/10.3310/AQXC8219
7. https://www.researchgate.net/publication/337402647

58. Advancements in Diabetes Management and Cardiovascular Health

Antonio Ceriello

ABSTRACT

- In most of the intervention studies in settings of T2D, a reduction in the magnitude of diverse CV risk factors have translated into tangible benefits on hard endpoints.
- On the other side, no trial has clearly proven that a reduction in variability per se, independently of the risk factor magnitude, is beneficial. However, evidence is growing suggesting that the variability of a risk factor might be not less dangerous than its magnitude and/or the time spent having it in an abnormal level.
- Moreover, it is also enough clear that the variability of each factor is additive in leading to the final picture of a diabetic complication.
- Therefore, from a therapeutic viewpoint, is it time to try to reduce both magnitude and variability of CV risk factors?
- Because an improvement of the quality of care and the attainment of their target seem to be the best strategy to reach this goal, we believe that the answer is not complicated.

59. D-Genius Symposium (Feb 13th 2PM: Diabetes India Hall) Common yet Underrated Challenges in Daily Diabetes Therapy

Praveen Gangadhara

ABSTRACT

The management of diabetes in India poses a unique and complex challenges due to high burden of the disease. Individuals known to have diabetes represent the tip of the iceberg, as an equal or even larger number of patients have undiagnosed diabetes.[1] The prevalence of diabetes and other metabolic NCDs in India is considerably higher than previously estimated.[2] Despite advancement in different classes of oral and injectable therapies for treatment of type 2 diabetes (T2DM) over the last decade, glycemic control is suboptimal leading to increased risk of complications. Clinical inertia, poor drug adherence, low disease awareness, regular follow-up, use of technology are crucial challenges for achieving glycaemic targets especially in the real-world clinical setting.[3]

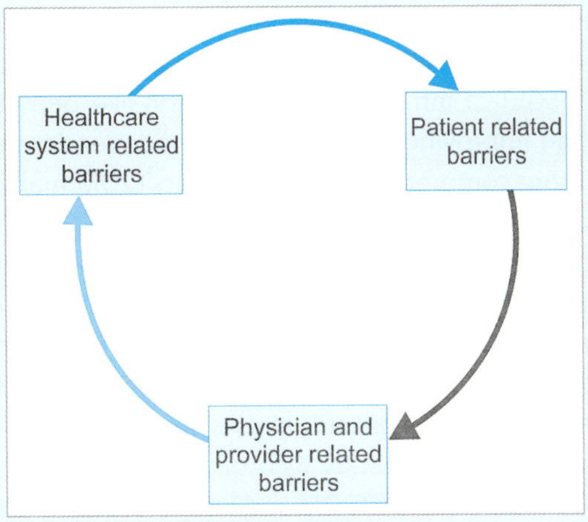

Some of the common yet under-rated challenges in our country includes:

1. Precision therapy versus Personalised therapy
2. Importance of Time in Range (TIR) along with HbA1c control, minimizing risk of hypoglycaemic especially nocturnal hypoglycaemic
3. Treatment addressing our dietary habits: High carbohydrate diets and higher glycaemic response in Asian Indians
4. Use of technology in the management of diabetes
5. Access to quality medications/injectables and standard of care.

Addressing these challenges requires a multifaceted approach involving healthcare providers, policy makers, patient support organizations, pharmaceutical industry to deliver standard of care and achieve desired glycaemic control.

REFERENCES

1. Mathur P, Leburu S, Kulothungan V. Prevalence, Awareness, Treatment and Control of Diabetes in India From the Countrywide National NCD Monitoring Survey. Front Public Health. 2022;10:748157.
2. Anjana RM, Unnikrishnan R, Deepa M, et al. Metabolic non-communicable disease health report of India: the ICMR-INDIAB national cross-sectional study (ICMR-INDIAB-17). Lancet Diabetes Endocrinol. 2023;11(7):474-489.
3. Borgharkar SS, Das SS. Real-world evidence of glycemic control among patients with type 2 diabetes mellitus in India: the TIGHT study. BMJ Open Diabetes Res Care. 2019;7(1):e000654.

60. Current Goals in T2DM: Is Glycemic Control Enough?

Ami Sanghvi

ABSTRACT

The management of type 2 diabetes mellitus (T2DM) has long centered on glycemic control as a cornerstone of treatment. This approach is grounded in robust evidence demonstrating that maintaining hemoglobin A1c (HbA1c) levels below 7% significantly reduces the risk of microvascular complications such as retinopathy, nephropathy, and neuropathy.[1] However, emerging research has challenged the adequacy of glycemic control as the sole focus, emphasizing the need for a broader approach to managing T2DM.

Macrovascular complications, including cardiovascular disease (CVD), remain the leading cause of mortality in T2DM patients. Landmark trials, such as EMPA-REG OUTCOME[2] and the LEADER trial,[3] have highlighted the benefits of sodium-glucose cotransporter-2 (SGLT-2) inhibitors and glucagon-like peptide-1 receptor agonists (GLP-1 RAs) in reducing cardiovascular events and improving renal outcomes, independent of glycemic control. These findings suggest a paradigm shift toward a more comprehensive approach to T2DM management, prioritizing cardiovascular and renal protection alongside glucose regulation.

Additionally, patient-centric goals, including weight management, minimizing hypoglycemia risk, and improving quality of life, are increasingly recognized as critical components of care. Obesity, a major contributor to T2DM pathogenesis, is now addressed with pharmacological options such as GLP-1 RAs, which offer both glycemic and weight-reduction benefits.

This talk explores the evolving goals in T2DM management, underscoring the inadequacy of glycemic control alone. It advocates for integrated strategies targeting multifactorial risks, incorporating lifestyle interventions, individualized pharmacotherapy, and addressing patient-specific needs. By broadening the scope of treatment objectives, healthcare providers can more effectively reduce the burden of T2DM and improve long-term outcomes.

REFERENCES

1. UK Prospective Diabetes Study (UKPDS) Group. Intensive blood-glucose control with sulphonylureas or insulin compared with conventional treatment and risk of complications in patients with type 2 diabetes. Lancet. 1998;352(9131):837-53.
2. Zinman, B, Wanner C, Lachin JM, Fitchett D, Bluhmki E, Hantel S, et al. Empagliflozin, cardiovascular outcomes, and mortality in type 2 diabetes. N Engl J Med. 2015;373(22):2117-28.
3. Marso SP, Daniels GH, Brown-Frandsen K, Kristensen P, Mann JFE, Nauck MA, et al. Liraglutide and cardiovascular outcomes in type 2 diabetes. N Engl J Med. 2016;375(4):311-22.

61. Sarcopenia and Diabetes

Anubha Srivastava, Jayant Agarwal

ABSTRACT

Introduction: Sarcopenia—"sarx" meaning flesh and "penia" meaning loss is Greek word and was first coined by Rosenberg et al. in 1989. Primary Sarcopenia affects older individuals due to age-related muscular atrophy. Systemic ailments that affects muscles lead to Secondary Sarcopenia. International Classification of illness (ICD-10) has given it as code M 62.84.[1] Diabetes and Sarcopenia are both common in Elderly and are interrelated. The occurrence rate of Sarcopenia in T2DM is 15 to 44%.[2] The risk factors of sarcopenia are aging, malnutrition lack of physical activity, chronic condition like diabetes. Sarcopenia is an emerging public health issue in elderly diabetics and is defined as age related progressive muscle mass loss and muscle function and physical performance which results in frailty, disability, falls, fractures and hospitalisation. Major mechanisms by which diabetes causes sarcopenia are increased insulin resistance, advanced glycation end products, chronic inflammation and oxidative stress.

The three dynamic approaches by measuring changes in:

1. Muscle strength (handgrip strength)
2. Physical performance (usual gait speed)
3. Appendicular skeletal muscle mass (ASM)

Conclusion: T2DM and sarcopenia are closely associated with one another. Muscle health impairment may contribute to progression of T2DM. Management should be individualised to patients from selection of oral hypoglycaemic agents to specific exercises and protein-rich nutrition.

REFERENCES

1. Cao L, Morley JE. Sarcopenia Is Recognized as an Independent Condition by an International Classification of Disease, Tenth Revision, Clinical Modification (ICD-10-CM) Code. J. Am. Med. Dir. Assoc. 2016;17:675-7.
2. Chen LK, Woo J, Assanta chai P, Auyeung TW, Chou MY, Iijima K, et al. Asian Working Group for Sarcopenia: 2019 Consensus Update on Sarcopenia Diagnosis and Treatment. J. Am. Med. Dir. Assoc. 2020;21:300-7.e2.

62. Beyond the Numbers: Understanding and Addressing Diabetes Distress in Clinical Practice

Alka Chadha

ABSTRACT

When we talk about managing diabetes, the conversation often revolves around numbers—blood glucose levels, HbA1c targets, insulin doses. But behind those numbers lies something deeply personal: The *emotional weight* of living with diabetes every single day.

Diabetes distress isn't the same as depression. It is the unique emotional exhaustion that comes from the relentless demands of managing diabetes—monitoring blood sugar, making food choices, staying physically active, managing medications, and dealing with the fear of complications. It's a weight that can silently impact self-care, health outcomes, and overall well-being.

In this talk, we'll explore:

- **What diabetes distress looks like** and how it differs from depression.
- **How to identify it early** using tools like the **Problem Areas in Diabetes (PAID)** scale and the **Diabetes Distress Scale (DDS)**.
- **How to create a safe space** where patients feel comfortable sharing their emotional struggles.

We'll discuss simple yet powerful ways healthcare providers can go beyond clinical markers and make emotional well-being a routine part of diabetes care.

Through real-life stories, practical strategies, and easy-to-apply tools, this session will highlight the importance of building trust, having honest conversations, and working *with* patients—not just *on* patients—to set achievable goals.

When we address diabetes distress with compassion and intention, we're not just improving numbers—we're improving lives.

Let's go *beyond the numbers* and bring humanity back into diabetes care.

63. Asymptomatic Bacteriuria in Females Suffering from Type 2 Diabetes Mellitus

Abha Gupta

ABSTRACT

Type 2 diabetes mellitus is a heterogeneous group of disorders characterized by variable degree of insulin resistance, impaired insulin secretion, and increased glucose production. Clinical features include polydipsia, polyuria and weight loss. Long term hyperglycemia will lead to organ dysfunction including vision loss, renal failure, cardiovascular disease, sexual dysfunction, gastrointestinal and urinary tract infections.

High glucose concentration in urine promotes urinary colonisation of microorganisms and the patient becomes more prone to microvascular disease of the kidneys. The human body's ability to fight pathogens decreases, the patient's urethral mucosal defence barrier function decreases, and pathogens are more likely to invade, increasing the risk of urinary infections.

The definition of a symptomatic bacteria (ASB) used in many studies refers to the presence of a freshly voided midstream urine specimen yielding positive cultures ($\geq 10^5$ CFU/mL) of the same bacterium in a patient without symptoms of urinary tract infection such as dysuria urgency urinary frequency or fever.

The urethra of women is short, close to the anus and the colonisation rate of pathogens around the urethra is high. The glycogen content of vaginal epithelium decreases due to diabetes, the pH value increases, the ecological environment of vaginal lactic acid bacteria is destroyed, the flora is unbalanced and it is easily infected. The most common bacteria that causing ASB isolated from both diabetic patients and non diabetics are *E. Coli, Klebsiella* species, *Staphylococcus saprophyticus*, *Staphylococcus aureus* and *Candida albicans*.

ASB is found to be three to four times more common in in women with diabetes than in healthy women. The bacteriuric patients with worse baseline HbA1c values were at greater risk of UTI. The presence of ASB may be considered a risk factor for subsequent symptomatic UTI on follow up but has no adverse effect on kidney function.

Two consecutive urine cultures should be performed to confirm the persistence of bacteriuria before making the diagnosis of asymptomatic bacteriuria and two voided specimens with $\geq$100,000 (10^5) CFU/mL indicating presence of same organism are needed to predict bladder bacteriuria.

Most patients with asymptomatic bacteriuria have no adverse consequences and derive no benefit from antibiotic therapy. Therefore, treatment of ASB is not routinely recommended except in case of pregnant females, neurogenic bladder and renal transplant, which warrants screening and treatment.

64. Role of Family Dynamics in Managing Diabetes Related Mental Health

Saritha Kakani

ABSTRACT

Family support plays a pivotal role in mitigating the emotional impact of diabetes. This involves providing emotional reassurance and understanding to individuals navigating the complexities of diabetes. Family members who offer empathy and support contribute significantly to the emotional well-being of their loved ones with diabetes.

Diabetes self-management education (DSME) is a critical component of care for all individuals with diabetes.[1] Involving family in self-care interventions may positively influence patients' diabetes outcomes as well as have a positive impact on their emotional well-being. Family members can often share the responsibility of diabetes management. They can provide many forms of support, such as driving patients to appointments or helping inject insulin and providing social and emotional support in helping patients cope with their disease.[2,3] Through their communications and attitudes, family members often have a significant impact on a patient's psychological well-being, decision to follow recommendations for medical treatment, and ability to initiate and maintain changes in diet and exercise.[4]

III. Assessment of patient's social support

Positive family environment has warmth and closeness—good metabolic control

Negative family environment has conflict and criticism—poor metabolic control

DE should assess the family involvement with respect to:

- Reminding about treatment recommendations
- Family accompanying for check-ups
- Supporting dietary modifications
- Helping financially
- Providing encouragement

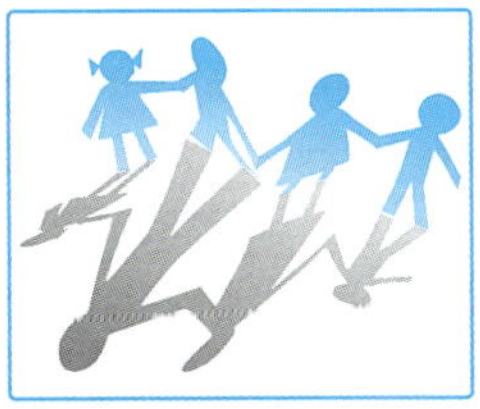

The chronic nature of diabetes introduces a substantial emotional burden on individuals and their families. The constant need for self-management, concerns about potential complications, and the unpredictability of blood glucose levels contribute to heightened stress, anxiety, and in some cases, depression. The emotional dimensions of diabetes significantly impact individuals and reverberate throughout the family unit, necessitating a subtle understanding of emotional support and coping strategies. In response to the emotional challenges posed by diabetes, families often develop coping strategies to foster resilience. By understanding and promoting effective coping strategies, families can contribute significantly to the overall mental health of their members living with diabetes.

REFERENCES

1. ADA. Standards of medical care in diabetes--2014. Diabetes Care. 2014:37 Suppl 1:S14-80.
2. Fisher L, Chesla CA, Bartz RJ, Gilliss C, Skaff MA, Sabogal F, et al. The family and type 2 diabetes: framework for intervention. Diabetes Educ. 1998;24:599-607.
3. Wagner EH, Austin BT, Davis C, Hindmarsh M, Schaefer J, Bonomi A. Improving chronic illness care: translating evidence into action. . Health Aff (Millwood). 2001;20(6):64-78.
4. Burg M, Seeman T. Families and health: The negative side of social ties. Annals of Behavioral Medicine. 1994;46:1097-108.

65. Postpartum Care for the Women with HIP

Swari Srivastava

ABSTRACT

Gestational diabetes mellitus (GDM) presents significant risks for both mothers and infants. With over 50% of women diagnosed with GDM expected to develop type 2 diabetes mellitus (T2DM) later in life, conducting postpartum oral glucose tolerance testing (OGTT) is critical for initiating suitable lifestyle interventions and pharmacological treatments.

Less than 50% of women with GDM complete postpartum OGTT, this being more often with women with limited education, restricted access to healthcare. Evidence indicates that current healthcare systems often lose patients during the postpartum transition from pregnancy-specific care to primary care.

Long-term management for women with GDM includes postpartum glucose tolerance testing. Organizations such as ACOG and ADA recommend that women with GDM receive follow-up care 6–12 weeks postpartum to assess blood pressure, body mass index (BMI), and metabolic health, in addition to addressing routine postpartum concerns. Furthermore, women are advised to visit their primary care providers within a year of delivery. During these visits, primary care providers can conduct additional metabolic assessments, prescribe pharmacologic therapies, and promote lifestyle interventions such as weight loss, which has been shown to significantly reduce diabetes risk, as evidenced by the Diabetes Prevention Program.

Previous research has highlighted strategies to improve OGTT completion rates for T2DM prevention. Proposed best practices include:

A. Providing enhanced support to help patients identify long-term healthcare providers
B. Implementing test reminders for both patients and providers
C. Formalizing communication between obstetricians and primary care providers.

Further studies are warranted to refine and validate these multi-faceted approaches for identifying and mitigating diabetes risk.

REFERENCE

1. Martinez NG, Niznik CM, Yee LM. Optimizing postpartum care for the patient with gestational diabetes mellitus. Am J Obstet Gynecol. 2017; 217(3):314-21.

66. Should Periodontal Therapy be Standardized as Part of Diabetes Management Plans?

Priya Phatak

ABSTRACT

Periodontal disease and diabetes share a two-way relationship.[1] It is not just an oral health issue—it contributes to the systemic manifestations of diabetes and is considered the sixth complication of diabetes. [2]

Periodontitis is an infection, and the bacteria from our gums enter the bloodstream, creating a systemic inflammatory response and an increased risk for systemic diseases like diabetes and cardiovascular diseases.[3] It can cause pain, discomfort, and difficulty chewing, negatively impacting nutrition and overall well-being. Scaling, root planing, and proper oral care can reduce bacterial load and systemic inflammation.

International health organizations, including the American Diabetes Association (ADA) and the World Health Organization (WHO), have recognized the bidirectional relationship between periodontal disease and diabetes. The ADA emphasizes the importance of periodontal care in a comprehensive diabetes management plan. As we move toward personalized care, integrating periodontal therapy is not just beneficial—it is essential.[4]

Managing both periodontal health and diabetes together can significantly improve a person's overall health and quality of life. Periodontal therapy is minimally invasive and has no side effects or downside. Even in patients who are borderline diabetic or have no periodontal manifestations so far, there is no harm plus, it will prevent future complications.

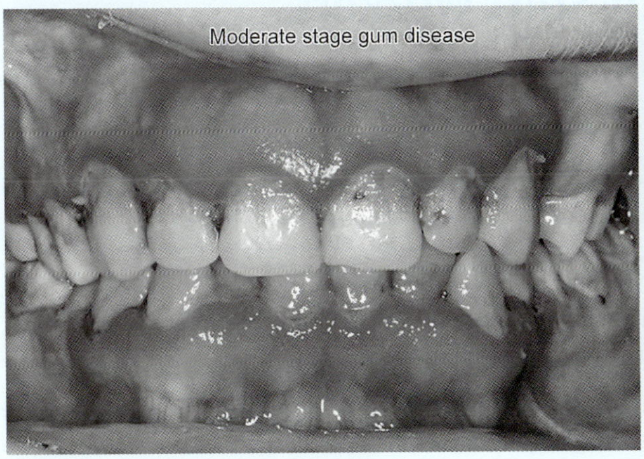

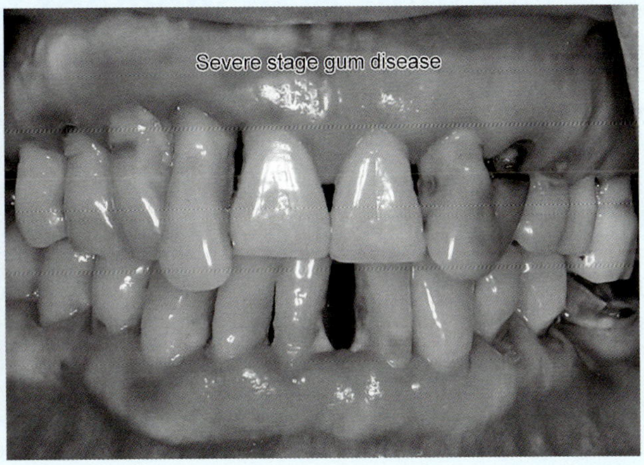

For color version (see color plate).

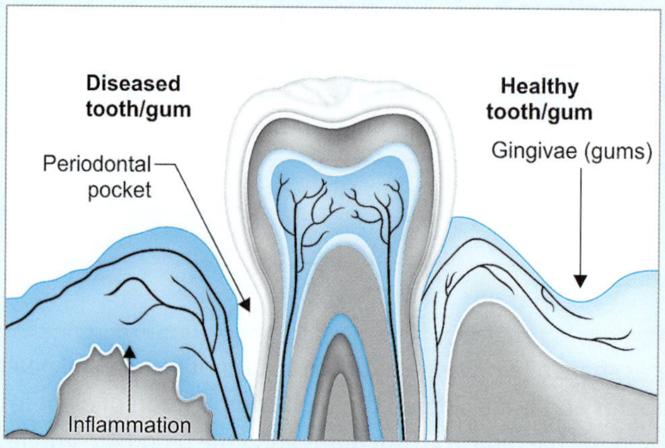

REFERENCES

1. Preshaw PM, Alba AL, Herrera D, et al. Periodontitis and diabetes: a two-way relationship. Diabetologia. 2012;55(1):21-31.
2. Harald Löe. Periodontal Disease: The sixth complication of diabetes mellitus. Diabetes Care. 1993;16(1):329-334.
3. Kim J, Amar S. Periodontal disease and systemic conditions: a bidirectional relationship. Odontology. 2006;94(1):10-21.
4. Online Available From https://diabetes.org/health-wellness/keeping-your-mouth-healthy

67. Focus on the Clock, Triumphs and Challenges in Diabetes Management for Shift Workers

Sandeep Suri

ABSTRACT

Shift workers, especially those with diabetes, face unique challenges in managing their condition due to disruptions in their circadian rhythms and irregular eating, sleeping, and activity patterns. From an endocrinologist's perspective, these factors can significantly impact glucose control, insulin sensitivity, and overall metabolic health.

Triumphs: Advances in diabetes technology, such as continuous glucose monitors (CGMs) and insulin pumps, have been transformative in helping shift workers maintain better glucose control. These tools provide real-time data and allow for more flexible insulin adjustments, making it easier for individuals to respond to changing schedules. Additionally, education on carbohydrate counting, appropriate insulin dosages, and lifestyle modifications tailored to shift work can empower patients to manage their diabetes effectively.

Challenges: The most significant challenge is the misalignment between the body's internal clock and external environment. Shift work, especially night shifts, can disrupt the secretion of insulin and other hormones, leading to insulin resistance and unpredictable blood sugar fluctuations. Irregular meal times and poor sleep can exacerbate this. For instance, late-night eating or eating heavy meals before sleep can spike blood glucose levels. Moreover, sleep deprivation, a common issue among shift workers, can impair glucose metabolism and insulin action, further complicating management.

Also, the social and psychological aspects of shift work—such as stress, fatigue, and limited access to healthy food options—can negatively affect adherence to treatment regimens. Managing diabetes during irregular hours requires personalized care plans, continuous monitoring, and support for lifestyle changes to minimize long-term complications.

In conclusion, while modern technology offers promising solutions, managing diabetes as a shift worker remains complex, requiring ongoing adjustments and a multidisciplinary approach to care.

68. Simplifying Diabetes Management in Primary Care: New Algorithms for Treatment Decision-making

Kannan Natarajan

ABSTRACT

Diabetes mellitus, a chronic metabolic disorder marked by elevated blood glucose levels, poses a significant risk for complications, including cardiovascular, renal, and neurological damage. The American Diabetes Association (ADA) 2023 guidelines emphasize an updated approach to screening, prevention, and management of type 2 diabetes.

Effective management begins with early screening and accurate diagnosis of prediabetes and diabetes, followed by interventions aimed at preventing disease progression. The guidelines advocate the use of continuous glucose monitoring (CGM) to standardize glucose assessment metrics and refine glycaemic target evaluation.

Non-pharmacological interventions, including lifestyle modifications, remain integral to treatment. For pharmacological management, the ADA proposes a patient-centred approach emphasizing cardiorenal protection and weight management. Metformin retains its position as the first-line therapy unless contraindicated. Early combination therapy is encouraged for patients with high HbA1c (>8.5%). For patients with atherosclerotic cardiovascular disease (ASCVD), heart failure (HF), or chronic kidney disease (CKD), SGLT2 inhibitors and GLP-1 receptor agonists are recommended due to their proven cardiorenal benefits. Additionally, weight-neutral or weight-reducing medications are prioritized for patients with obesity, and agents like DPP-4 inhibitors are favoured for minimizing hypoglycaemia risk.

The ADA introduces a simplified, stepwise treatment algorithm. Therapy is tailored based on patient comorbidities, with adjustments every 3–6 months to meet glycaemic targets. To support implementation in primary care, emphasis is placed on team education, shared decision-making, technology integration, and regular screening for diabetes complications.

Emerging recommendations extend to type 2 diabetes in youth, focusing on obesity prevention. The guidelines underscore the importance of primary care teams in adopting these evidence-based strategies to improve diabetes outcomes effectively.

69. Measuring Outcomes of DSMEs

Tatjana Milenkovic

ABSTRACT

Faculty of Medicine, Ss. Cyril and Methodius University in Skopje, Macedonia; University Clinic for endocrinology, diabetes and metabolic disorders, Diabetes Self-Management Education (DSME) is a cornerstone in improving health outcomes for individuals with diabetes. Measuring the outcomes of DSME programs is essential to assess their effectiveness and inform continuous improvement. Methods and metrics for evaluating DSME outcomes are focusing on clinical, behavioral, and psychosocial dimensions. Clinical outcomes, such as HbA1c levels, blood pressure, and lipid profiles, are widely used to assess the physiological impact of DSME. Behavioral outcomes, including medication adherence, dietary changes, and physical activity levels, reflect the program's influence on patients' daily self-management practices. Psychosocial outcomes, such as diabetes-related distress, self-efficacy, and quality of life, provide insights into the emotional and psychological benefits of DSME.

Evaluation methods include both quantitative and qualitative approaches, including pre-and post-program surveys, focus groups, and longitudinal tracking. Standardized tools like the Diabetes Self-Management Questionnaire (DSMQ) and Patient-Reported Outcome Measures (PROMs) are engaged to ensure consistency and comparability. Key findings indicate that structured DSME programs lead to significant improvements in glycemic control, enhanced self-care behaviors, and reduced diabetes-related distress. However, challenges remain in capturing long-term outcomes, addressing individual variability, and integrating assessments into routine clinical practice.

There is the need for a multidimensional and patient-centered approach to measure DSME outcomes effectively. Emphasizing tailored interventions and leveraging digital health tools can further enhance the reach and impact of DSME programs. Future research should focus on standardizing metrics and exploring innovative strategies to ensure sustainable improvements in diabetes care and self-management.

70. Engagement of People With Diabetes and Coaching Models. Albanian Example of Group Education

Florian Toti, Adriana Lapardhaja, Evis Sinjari, Marilda Hysa, Luftime Bruka

ABSTRACT

Diabetes has reached epidemic proportions in most countries. The incidence of diabetes is expected to double worldwide in the next twenty years. The economic costs of diabetes are huge and are doubled by the onset of complications resulting from poor disease control.

Several major randomized controlled trials (RCTs) have shown reduction of complications with more intensive pharmacotherapy for hypertension, dyslipidemia and hyperglycemia in type 2 diabetes (T2D). A range of self-management interventions focusing on patient education and empowerment have also been shown to be effective.

Coaching model is a pragmatic intervention that primes the patient to self-manage by adhering to medication and make relevant behavior changes. It also, importantly, encourages patients to take greater initiative in the therapeutic alliance, which enables treatment to be appropriately intensified according to clinical practice guidelines in order to achieve treatment goals.

50 PWD were recruited for this study. During a six-month period, a monthly group session was held with diabetic patients. A diabetologist, and a nurse were participating as facilitator and educators during the sessions. In every education session from the group was decided the program for the next appointment. HbA1c, lipid profile and anthropometric measurements has been completed at the beginning, at 3 and 6 months, as well questions about psycho-emotional state and satisfaction with diabetes treatment. The results were compared for the same periods.

Results: From 50, 47 (94%) of the patients completed the 6 months education program. Mean HbA1c decreased from 8.43 ± 1.09% to 7.74 ± 1.07% ($p < 0.05$), mean weight 82.54 ± 20.8 kg versus 80.47 ± 20.11 kg ($p < 0.05$). The patients had a slight increase in HDL cholesterol 54.7 ± 7.65 mg/dL to 59.05 ± 7.29 mg/dL. Their overall satisfaction with diabetes treatment improved from 35 to 56% ($p < 0.01$).

Therapeutic education should be integrated part of diabetes treatment and weight control. Empowering diabetic patients not only affect in a positive way their general well-being, and metabolic control, but improve their confidence in self-efficacy and satisfaction with treatment. Group education facilitates patients' active participation, and is less time consuming.

71. Targeting Glycaemic Levels in GDM: How Tight is Tight Enough?

P Popova

ABSTRACT

Optimal glycaemic targets for the treatment of gestational diabetes mellitus (GDM) have not been universally defined. There is wide variation in recommendations for glycaemic targets. Until recently, there were no data from randomised controlled trials (RCTs) designed to define optimal treatment targets.

Observational studies in normal pregnancy show that normal glucose levels are significantly lower than the targets currently recommended for the management of GDM.

Two RCTs with different intensities of glycaemic control have recently been completed. C Crowther's cluster-randomised trial of more than 1,000 women produced conflicting results. There was no effect of glycaemic targets on the primary outcome of LGA babies. However, the study did show a reduction in the composite of major neonatal health outcomes and an increase in major maternal health outcomes. There was an increased need for pharmacological treatment in the tighter target group.

In our RCT at the Almazov Centre, 650 women with GDM were randomised. Group 1 were recommended tighter glycaemic targets in line with current Russian guidelines (fasting blood glucose <5.1 and <7.0 mmol/L 1 hour postprandial). Group 2 was recommended less stringent glycaemic targets, which are currently supported by ADA and FIGO.

Our study showed benefits of tighter targets for the primary outcome. There was a reduction in the proportion of LGA in the tighter target group. However, this required increased use of insulin therapy. And there was no difference in the secondary outcomes for both mothers and babies. Another potential benefit of tighter targets for offspring metabolic health was a reduction in the leptin/adiponectin ratio in cord blood.

Thus, tighter glycaemic targets are beneficial for the infant (based on two RCTs) and are unlikely to result in any difference in maternal morbidity.

72. Practical Aspects of Insulin Therapy: Clinical Tips on Techniques—Store, Site and Rotation

Sudhir Chandra Jha

ABSTRACT

Diabetes affects 537 million people between the ages of 20 and 79 years, or 10.5% of the population, making it a global health concern. Managing type 1 and type 2 diabetes, controlling blood sugar levels, minimising complications, and enhancing quality of life all depend on effective insulin therapy. Precise technique, site selection, and rotation are necessary for effective insulin administration. Important therapeutic recommendations for effective insulin therapy is highlighted in this abstract.

Among the various forms of insulin, including rapid-acting, short-acting, intermediate-acting, and long-acting insulin, it is crucial to choose the appropriate type based on one's needs and store them appropriately. The next important stage in the insulin administration process is selecting the right equipment from the variety of options available, such as insulin pens, syringes, and pumps. Typical injection locations are the abdomen, thighs, upper arms, and buttocks. Proper injection procedures involve the right needle depth and angle, which means that the needle should be inserted in the subcutaneous tissue without touching the muscle tissue at a 90° angle for people of normal weight or at a 45° angle for very thin patients. Rotating injection sites on a regular basis guarantees uniform absorption and prevents lipo-hypertrophy. Lipo-hypertrophy causes blood glucose levels to become unstable by decreasing insulin absorption. A regular rotation pattern can help prevent problems at the injection site. Structured rotation, which includes rotation between injection sites as well as inside them, is advised. Educating patients on self-monitoring, identifying hypoglycaemia and hyperglycaemia and knowing when to seek medical attention is essential for successful insulin therapy. By using the right method, site selection, and rotation, medical professionals can increase the effectiveness of insulin therapy and lower the chance of negative consequences. Patients can improve their quality of life and attain optimal glycaemic management by putting these useful recommendations into practice.

73. Recognizing and Addressing Foot Care in Diabetes: Practical Tips

Sandeep Rai

ABSTRACT

Diabetic foot ulcers (DFU) are a preventable complication in adults with diabetes. Every twenty seconds, a limb is lost in the world due to diabetic foot. A triad of neuropathy, arterial occlusive disease along with trauma and secondary infection account for the pathophysiology of diabetic foot ulcer. High risk foot can be assessed by enquiring about factors such as bare foot walking, diabetic neuropathy with loss of protective sensation, symptoms of PAD, foot deformity, poor glycemic control, smoking and visual impairment. Tests performed to identify patients of, at risk foot, include 10 g monofilament to assess neuropathy in diabetic patients. Using the tuning fork is an easy and inexpensive way to test vibratory sensation. A biothesiometer measures the Vibration Perception Threshold (VPT).There are devices which identify high plantar pressure including mats to measure barefoot plantar pressure. Ankle brachial pressure index is the most common method used to screen patients for presence of peripheral artery disease. Toe pressure and Toe Brachial Index (TBI) may provide a more reliable assessment of perfusion. Color duplex ultrasound and angiography (MRA) can be done to assess patients with peripheral arterial disease. Laser Doppler Flowmetry is being used nowadays to measure the local microcirculatory blood perfusion.

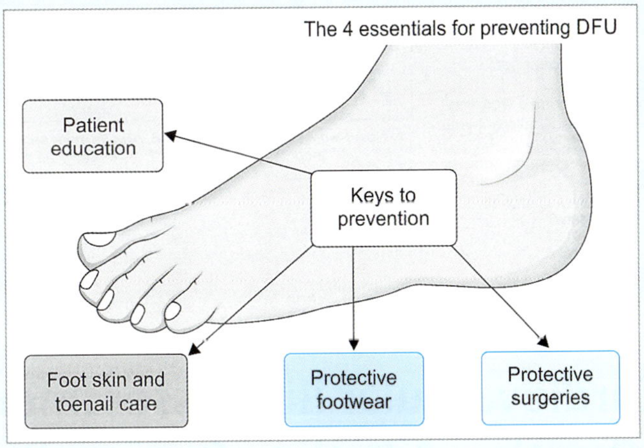

Few practical tips that can be given to Diabetes patients coming to clinics and hospitals are—Check your feet every day for cuts, redness, swelling, sores, blisters, corns, or calluses. Wash your feet every day in warm (not hot) water and ensure they are thoroughly dried. Avoid placing your feet too close to radiant heaters. Never walk barefoot, even inside house. Wear shoes that fit well and always wear socks without seams. Cut your toenails straight across and smooth out any sharp edges with a nail file. Don't try to remove corns or calluses yourself. Get your feet checked are at least once a year.

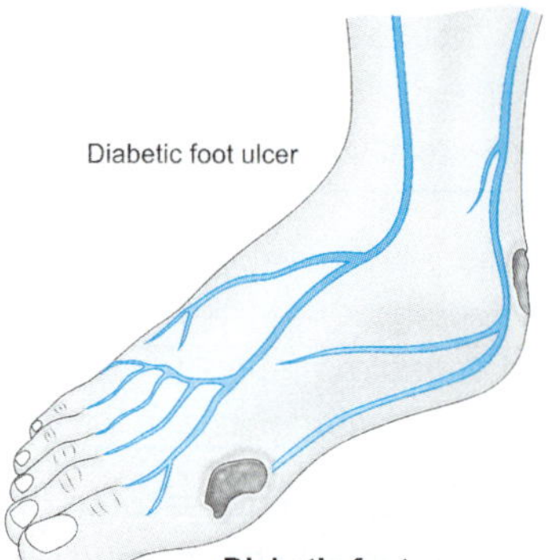

Diabetic foot

Inspect your feet daily. Check for cuts, blisters, redness, swelling, or nail problems. Use a magnifying hand mirror to look at the bottom of your feet. Call your doctor if you notice anything.
Wash your feet in lukewarm (not hot!) water. Keep your feet clean by washing them daily. But only use lukewarm water---the temperature you'd use on a newborn baby.
Be gentle when bathing your feet. Wash them using a soft washcloth or sponge. Dry by blotting or patting---and make sure to carefully dry between the toes.
Moisturize your feet—but not between your toes. Use a moisturizer daily to keep dry skin from itching or cracking. But DON'T moisturize between the toes-this could encourage a fungal infection.
Cut nails carefully—and straight across. Also, file the edges. Don't cut them too short, since this could lead to ingrown toe nails.
Never trim corns or calluses. No "bathroom surgery"---let your doctor do the job.
Wear clean, dry socks. Change them daily.
Avoid the wrong type of socks. Avoid tight elastic bands (they reduce circulation). Don't wear thick or bulky socks (they can fit poorly and irritate the skin).
Wear socks to bed. If your feet get cold at night, wear socks. NEVER use a heating pad or hot water bottle.
Shake out your shoes and inspect the inside before wearing. Remember, you may not feel a pebble---so always shake out your shoes before putting them on.
Keep your feet warm and dry. Don't get your feet wet in snow or rain. Wear warm socks and shoes in winter.
Never walk barefoot. Not even at home! You could step on something and get a scratch or cut.

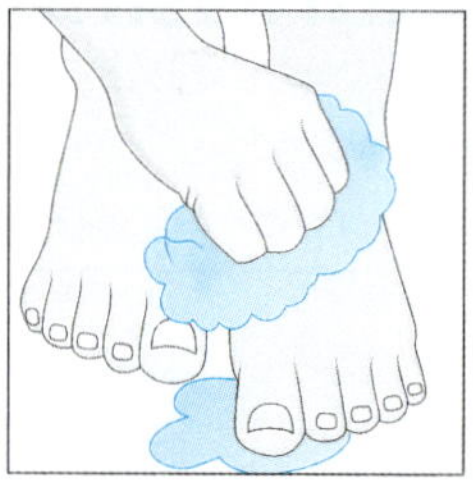
1. Wash your feet daily with lukewarm water soap, just as you wash your hands

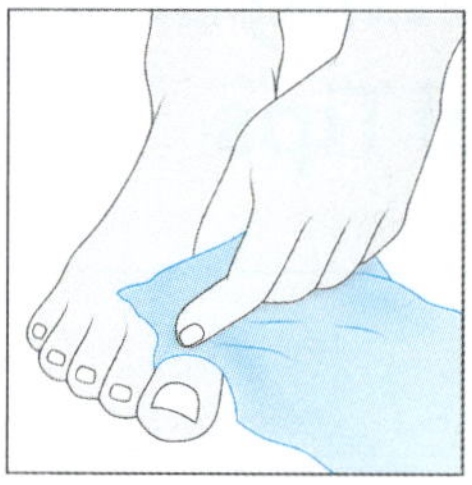
2. Dry your feet well, also between the toes,

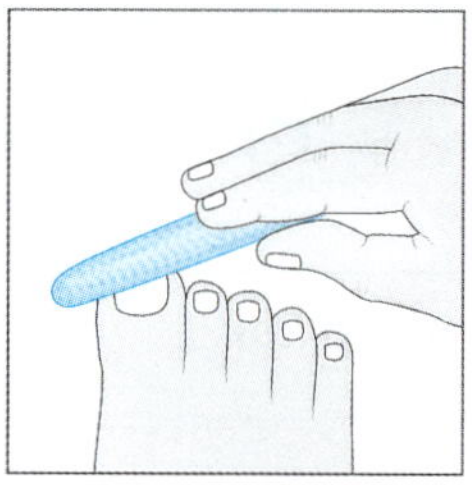
3. Use emery board to shape toenails even with ends of your toes.

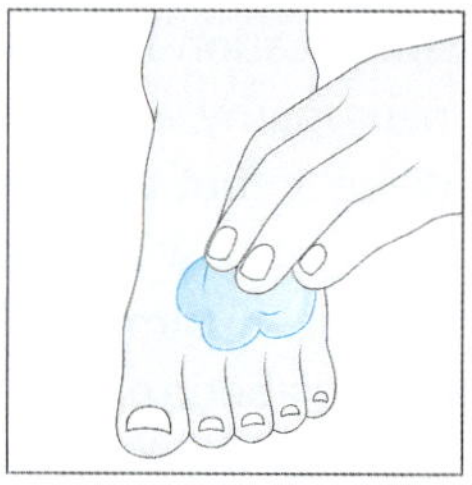
4. Keep the skin supple with a moisturizing lotion, but do not apply it between the toes

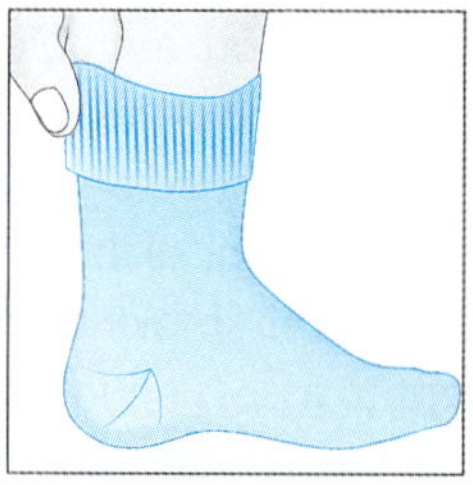
5. Change daily into clean, soft socks or stockings which must neither be too big nor too small.

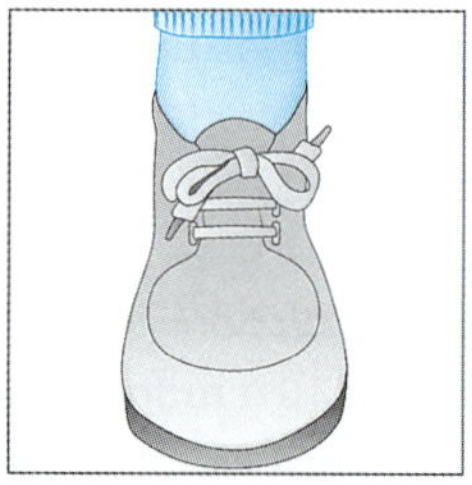
6. Keep your feet warm and dry preferably wear special padded socks and shoes of leather.

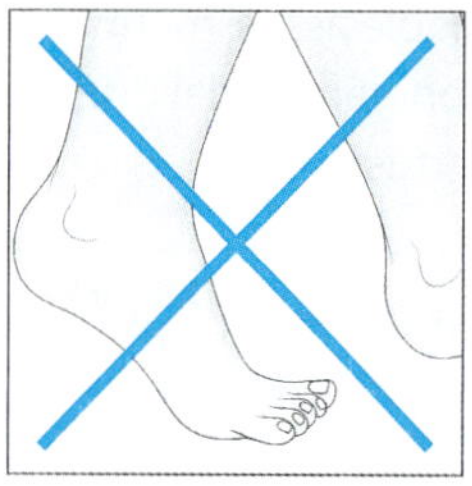
7. Never walk barefoot neither indoors nor outdoors

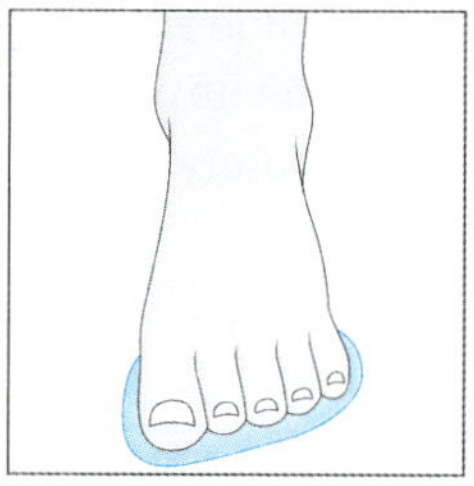
8. Always wear shoes that It this applies also to sandals

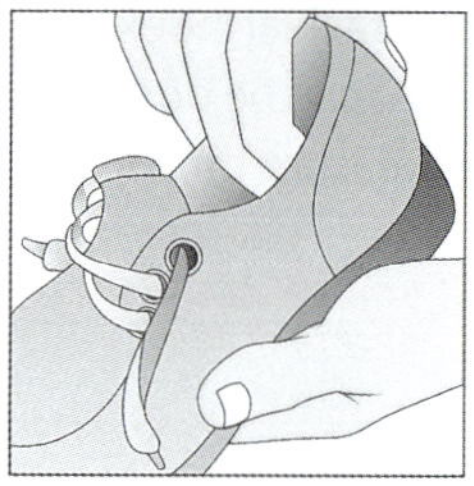
9. Examine your shoes every day for cracks, pebbles, nails, and other irregularities which may irritate the skin.

74. Refining Cardiovascular Risk Assessment in Diabetes in Clinical Practice: A Path to Personalized Care

Rajeev Chawla

ABSTRACT

Cardiovascular disease (CVD) remains the primary cause of morbidity and mortality in individuals with diabetes mellitus (DM), emphasizing the necessity for precise and individualized risk assessment. Traditional risk models, including the Framingham Risk Score, often underestimate the distinct and amplified cardiovascular risk in diabetic patients. Incorporating diabetes-specific factors—such as glycemic control, diabetes duration, and microvascular complications—alongside conventional risk factors enhances predictive accuracy and facilitates personalized care.

Advances in biomarkers like high-sensitivity C-reactive protein (hs-CRP) and imaging modalities such as coronary artery calcium (CAC) scoring have demonstrated significant potential in improving risk stratification. Additionally, emerging tools, such as genetic risk profiling and machine learning algorithms, provide a nuanced understanding of cardiovascular risk patterns by integrating complex datasets. Contemporary clinical guidelines increasingly recommend these advanced approaches to guide therapeutic decisions, such as the early initiation of statins, antihypertensives, and cardioprotective glucose-lowering agents, including SGLT2 inhibitors and GLP-1 receptor agonists.

Despite these developments, challenges persist in adopting enhanced risk assessment in routine practice, including financial constraints, limited access to advanced diagnostics, and integration complexities. Overcoming these barriers requires a multidisciplinary approach, improved clinical pathways, and enhanced provider education.

Refining cardiovascular risk assessment in diabetes is essential for reducing the burden of CVD and improving outcomes. Future research and innovation will play a pivotal role in bridging the gap between advanced risk prediction and effective prevention strategies, ultimately advancing personalized care in clinical practice.

REFERENCES

1. Grundy SM, Stone NJ, Bailey AL, et al. AHA/ACC guideline on the primary prevention of cardiovascular disease: 2019 update. Circulation. 2019;140:e596-646.
2. Arnett DK, Blumenthal RS, Albert MA, et al. ACC/AHA guideline on the primary prevention of cardiovascular disease: 2019. J Am Coll Cardiol. 2019;74(10):e177-232.
3. Rawshani A, Rawshani A, Franzén S, et al. Mortality and cardiovascular disease in type 1 and type 2 diabetes. N Engl J Med. 2017;376(15): 1407-18.
4. Cosentino F, Grant PJ, Aboyans V, et al. ESC guidelines on diabetes, pre-diabetes, and cardiovascular diseases developed in collaboration with the EASD. Eur Heart J. 2019;41(2):255-323.
5. Blaha MJ, Cainzos-Achirica M, Greenland P. Beyond traditional risk factors: Coronary artery calcium to guide a personalized approach to CVD prevention. J Am Coll Cardiol. 2021;77(24):3077-91.

75. Early Gestational Diabetes: Current Update

V Mohan

ABSTRACT

Gestational diabetes (GDM) refers to glucose intolerance first detected during pregnancy. Traditionally, GDM was diagnosed between 24–28 weeks of pregnancy. More recently, GDM is being diagnosed in the first trimester of pregnancy and this is referred to as 'Early GDM'.

The prevalence of eGDM varies widely due to different criteria being used. Women with eGDM present with a unique metabolic profile. The pathophysiology of eGDM appears to be worse beta-cell dysfunction compared to late GDM. Increased occurrence of adverse pregnancy outcomes, higher incidence of postpartum dysglycemia and a greater need for insulin use have been reported in women with eGDM. The **T**reatment **O**f **BO**oking **G**estational diabetes **M**ellitus (ToBOGM) study was the first large randomised control trial to show the benefits of treatment in women with eGDM in terms of better neonatal outcomes.

76. Role of Endothelial Dysfunction in Diabetic Erectile Dysfunction: A Therapeutic Target

Raveendran AV

ABSTRACT

The prevalence of erectile dysfunction (ED) is increasing worldwide. In people with diabetes, ED is the most common male sexual dysfunction. Diabetic erectile dysfunction (DED) is considered a special entity due to multifactorial etiology including vascular, hormonal, and neurological factors. ED is a local manifestation of a generalized atherosclerotic process in people with diabetes and endothelial dysfunction is the mother of all cardiovascular complications in diabetes. In simple words, endothelial dysfunction is defined as the abnormal or impaired response of the endothelial cells in the vascular wall to vasodilatory stimulus which promotes atherosclerosis. Endothelial cells play a key role in the production of nitric oxide (NO), which is important in the penile vasodilatation and erection. Inflammation, oxidative stress, impaired endothelial Nitric Oxide Synthase (eNOS) activity and reduced Nitric Oxide bioavailability plays a major role in the development of endothelial dysfunction in people with diabetes mellitus. Considering the central role of endothelial dysfunction in the development of DED, targeting the pathophysiological mechanism of endothelial dysfunction is a promising approach in the prevention and treatment of DED. Targeting endothelial dysfunction through lifestyle changes, pharmacological agents, or advanced therapies like gene or stem cell treatments is a promising approach for the treatment of DED. Reversal of endothelial dysfunction may be a target for future research.

Keywords: Diabetic erectile dysfunction, Endothelial dysfunction, Male sexual dysfunction.

6
Section

Complications and Comorbidities

77. Optimising CKD Care in People with Type 2 Diabetes Mellitus: Learnings from EMPA-KIDNEY Study

JJ Mukherjee

ABSTRACT

Chronic kidney disease (CKD) is a common complication of type 2 diabetes mellitus (T2DM). Effective management strategies, including dietary modifications and guideline directed blood glucose, blood pressure and serum lipids control are essential to prevent progression to ESRD. Among medications, the renin-angiotensin-aldosterone system (RAAS) blockers (ACEi/A2RB) are the first line agents that must be used, unless contraindicated, in all people with T2DM with CKD. The CREDENCE trial (Canagliflozin; 2019) firmly established the role of sodium-glucose co-transporter 2 inhibitors (SGLT2i) in reducing clinically relevant renal end-points in people with T2DM with CKD. The DAPA-CKD trial (Dapagliflozin; 2020) not only confirmed these findings but also extended the benefits to people with non-diabetic CKD.

The EMPA-KIDNEY trial (2022) was a phase 3, randomized, double-blind study designed to evaluate the efficacy and safety of empagliflozin in people with CKD, regardless of diabetes status. The trial enrolled 6609 people with moderate to severe CKD [eGFR: 20 to 45 mL/min/1.73 m^2, or 45 to 90 mL/min/1.73 m^2 with albuminuria ≥200 mg/g]. Participants were randomized to receive either empagliflozin (10 mg daily) or placebo; the primary endpoint was the first occurrence of a composite of kidney disease progression [progression to ESRD (initiation of maintenance dialysis or renal transplantation), sustained decrease of eGFR to < 10 mL/min/1.73 m^2, sustained eGFR decline ≥40%, or death from renal causes] or death from cardiovascular causes. Empagliflozin significantly reduced the primary end-point by 28% compared to placebo (hazard ratio 0.72, 95% CI 0.62–0.83, $p < 0.001$). Among the three secondary outcomes, empagliflozin showed a statistically significant reduction in hospitalization for any cause; however, the other two secondary endpoints (HHF/CVD and death from any cause), though numerically lesser in the empagliflozin group, failed to reach statistical significance. The benefits were observed in both diabetic and non-diabetic participants, as well as across all eGFR ranges studied. The most common side effects included mild volume depletion and genital infections. In conclusion, the EMPA-KIDNEY trial showed that among a wide range of people with CKD, treatment with empagliflozin led to a lower risk of progression of kidney disease or death from cardiovascular causes than placebo. This trial further expands the role of SGLT2i in the management of people with CKD.

78. A Practical Approach to a Person with Fatty Liver on Ultrasound

Rakesh M Parikh

ABSTRACT

Fatty liver detected on ultrasound is frequently associated with metabolic dysfunction-associated steatotic liver disease (MASLD), a condition encompassing a spectrum of liver injury linked to metabolic risk factors. Accurate risk stratification and timely intervention are essential to prevent progression to advanced fibrosis and cirrhosis.

The FIB-4 score, a non-invasive serum marker, serves as an effective initial tool to stratify patients based on their risk of advanced fibrosis. For those with indeterminate or elevated FIB-4 scores, transient elastography (FibroScan) provides valuable additional insights by assessing liver stiffness and identifying patients at significant risk.

Lifestyle modification is the cornerstone of MASLD management. Structured weight loss programs focusing on hypocaloric diets and increased physical activity have demonstrated substantial benefits, including reductions in hepatic steatosis, fibrosis risk, and cardiometabolic complications. Pharmacotherapy is indicated in select patients, particularly those with non-alcoholic steatohepatitis (NASH) or advanced fibrosis. Pioglitazone and vitamin E have shown efficacy in specific populations, while glucagon-like peptide-1 receptor agonists (GLP-1 RA) and sodium-glucose co-transporter-2 inhibitors (SGLT2i) offer promising results in patients with type 2 diabetes and metabolic syndrome. Recent therapeutic advancements include thyroid hormone receptor beta agonists, which target hepatic steatosis with favorable metabolic effects.

This approach underscores the importance of individualized care, combining non-invasive diagnostics with tailored interventions to optimize outcomes for patients with MASLD.

79. Diabetes and Lung: A Critical Association

Agam Vora

ABSTRACT

Diabetes mellitus (DM) and lung diseases share a significant yet often overlooked association, with serious implications for patient health. DM is known to compromise multiple organ systems, and the lungs are no exception. Individuals with diabetes are at a higher risk of developing tuberculosis (TB), with TB rates significantly elevated in this population. Furthermore, respiratory infections, which are among the leading global causes of mortality, tend to worsen in the presence of diabetes due to impaired immune function.

Lung function abnormalities, particularly restrictive defects, are frequently observed in individuals with poorly controlled diabetes. This is attributed to chronic hyperglycemia, which induces systemic inflammation, collagen glycation, and microvascular changes, adversely affecting pulmonary mechanics. Conversely, diabetes also complicates the management of chronic respiratory diseases, such as chronic obstructive pulmonary disease (COPD) and asthma, by worsening glycemic control and enhancing systemic inflammation.

The bidirectional impact of diabetes and lung diseases amplifies morbidity and mortality, causing far more damage than either condition in isolation. This interplay underscores the need for heightened vigilance in managing patients with either disease. All patients with respiratory conditions should be screened for diabetes, and similarly, diabetics must be evaluated for lung abnormalities, including infections like TB or obstructive conditions such as COPD.

Recognizing this harmful "friendship" between DM and lung diseases is crucial. Only by adopting a proactive approach can healthcare providers mitigate the compounded burden and improve outcomes for patients grappling with these intertwined conditions.

80. Holistic Cardio-Renal-Metabolic Care in T2DM: Optimizing Approach with SGLT2-i + DPP4-i Combination

Anant Nigam

ABSTRACT

There has been a paradigm shift in the management of T2 diabetes mellitus (T2DM). From just controlling glucose, the emphasis is now on a comprehensive approach to use therapies aimed at protecting the cardiovascular (i.e., heart failure, coronary artery disease, stroke and peripheral artery disease), renal (i.e., chronic kidney disease) and metabolic (i.e., obesity, metabolic associated fatty liver disease) (CVRM) complications. The focus is also to manage weight and minimize hypoglycemic risk. Early combination therapy in T2DM addresses multiple pathophysiologic defects, overcomes clinical inertia and thus enables a long and durable glycemic control. This helps in reducing the overall morbidity and mortality in T2DM.

The combination of a sodium-glucose co-transporter 2 inhibitor (SGLT-2i) and a Dipeptidyl peptidase-4 inhibitor (DPP-4i) is now considered vital because of their synergistic benefits in the holistic cardiorenal metabolic care in T2DM. Together, both classes effectively lower glucose. SGLT-2i decrease glucose reabsorption in the kidneys and promote urinary glucose excretion, while the DPP-4i increase insulin secretion and decrease glucagon levels in a glucose-dependent fashion. SGLT-2i help in weight loss and the DPP-4*is* are weight neutral. Together they support weight management and also have a low risk of hypoglycemia. Cardiovascular outcome trials (EMPA-REG, CANVAS, DECLARE), the dedicated kidney trials (CREDENCE, DAPA-CKD, EMPA-KIDNEY) and the heart-failure trials (EMPEROR-REDUCED, PRESERVED, DAPA-HF, DELIVER) with the SGLT-2*is* have shown significant cardio-renal benefits which include reduction of major cardiovascular events, prevention and treatment of heart failure. They lower urine-albumin creatinine ratio, and reduce kidney failure risk. The DPP-4*is* are cardiovascular safe, reduce albuminuria and thus can be used in chronic kidney disease. Thus the SGLT-2i+DPP-4i combination therapy is one of the best choices in the management of T2 DM.

81. Celiac Disease and Gluten Intolerance in Diabetic Patients: A Practical Approach

Warren Lee, Collip Hall

ABSTRACT

The published prevalence of celiac disease in Type 1 diabetes is 6–8% but some studies report higher prevalence in the region of 15–20% . It is important to diagnose Celiac Disease in diabetic patients because of potential effects on growth, glycemic variability and pubertal development as well as complication rates. The presenting symptoms can be mild—only being detected on routine screening , or moderate or severe. Ce D can present with lower HbA1c, sometimes severe hypoglycemia and lower insulin requirements and can present with immediate spikes of hyperglycemia or delayed and prolonged hyperglycemia, poor height growth, poor weight gain and delayed pubertal development and varying levels of insulin requirement as gluten intolerance can cause an acute rise in insulin resistance . Variability in insulin requirements may not be obvious in settings where gluten is taken with every meal, but In an Asian setting when gluten intake in any given meal may be high or nonexistent, hyperglycemia may follow a gluten-heavy meal with insulin doses optimized for a gluten light meal but hypoglycemia may follow a gluten-light meal with dosing optimized for a high gluten diet. Case finding strategies and case management are discussed: routine screening vs testing on clinical suspicion, CGMS based methods vs serological methods and whether biopsies are needed to confirm the diagnosis. I will discuss the practical aspects and pitfalls of attempting a gluten free diet and the role adjunctive probiotics and potential role of commercial enzyme preparations.

82. Novel Treatment Options in MASLD in Type 2 Diabetes Mellitus (T2DM)

Ashish Kumar

ABSTRACT

Metabolic dysfunction-associated steatotic liver disease (MASLD), a major cause of chronic liver disease, is closely associated with Type 2 Diabetes Mellitus (T2DM). T2DM exacerbates MASLD progression due to insulin resistance, chronic inflammation, and metabolic dysregulation, making effective treatment strategies essential. While lifestyle modifications remain the foundation, novel therapies are emerging that address both MASLD and T2DM.

Lifestyle Modifications: Weight loss of 7–10% through lifestyle changes significantly improves liver histology in MASLD. Caloric restriction combined with resistance or aerobic exercise not only reduces liver fat but also improves glycemic control in T2DM patients. Bariatric surgery is an option for selected individuals with severe obesity, offering substantial benefits for both MASLD and diabetes.

Pharmacological Therapies

Several drugs approved for T2DM management are showing promise in treating MASLD:

- GLP-1 Receptor Agonists (e.g., Semaglutide, Liraglutide): These drugs reduce steatosis and steatohepatitis via weight loss and insulin sensitivity improvements. Ongoing trials are exploring their potential to reduce liver fibrosis.
- SGLT2 Inhibitors (e.g., Empagliflozin): By improving insulin sensitivity and reducing hepatic fat accumulation, these drugs offer dual benefits for MASLD and T2DM.
- PPAR Agonists (e.g., Pioglitazone): Effective in improving both hepatic fibrosis and glycemic control, these drugs enhance adipose tissue function, mitigating insulin resistance.
- Dual GLP-1/GIP Agonists (e.g., Tirzepatide): Combining GLP-1 and GIP effects, these drugs provide significant weight loss and metabolic benefits, addressing both MASLD and T2DM.

Emerging Therapies: Agents such as resmetirom (THR-β agonist) and fibroblast growth factor 21 (FGF21) analogs show promise in improving MASLD outcomes but require further validation in T2DM populations.

Addressing MASLD in T2DM patients requires a multi-pronged approach combining lifestyle interventions and targeted therapies to mitigate disease progression and systemic complications.

Drug	Mechanism of action	Efficacy in MASLD with T2DM
GLP-1 Receptor Agonists (e.g., Semaglutide, Liraglutide)	Enhances insulin sensitivity, reduces appetite, promotes weight loss	Improves steatosis and steatohepatitis but limited impact on fibrosis regression
PPAR Agonists (e.g., Pioglitazone, Saroglitazar, Lanifibranor)	Modulates lipid metabolism, inflammation, and fibrosis	Improves fibrosis and steatohepatitis
SGLT2 Inhibitors (e.g., Empagliflozin, Dapagliflozin)	Reduces glucose reabsorption in the kidney, improves insulin sensitivity	Reduces liver fat and improves metabolic profile
Dual GLP-1/GIP Agonists (e.g., Tirzepatide)	Combines GLP-1 and GIP pathways for enhanced metabolic effects	Promising results in liver and metabolic health
Metformin	Improves insulin sensitivity	Limited evidence in improving liver histology but reduces HCC risk

83. Emerging Clinical and Real-World Evidence on AGI: Findings from Recent START AM Study

Debmalya Sanyal

ABSTRACT

Background and aim: Newly diagnosed type 2 diabetes (T2DM) patients in India oftenhave high HbA1c levels, majorly contributed by postprandial hyperglycemia (PPG) owing to high dietary carbohydrate intake. Majority of patients require combination of drugs with complimentary actions to achieve glycemic control. Timely initiation of therapy helps in early achievement of goals. Aim of the study was to assess the effectiveness and tolerability of acarbose-metformin fixed dose combination (FDC) in newly diagnosed T2DM patients who are eligible for dual therapy under real-life treatment condition.

Materials and methods: This was a prospective, observational, real-world study in newly diagnosed T2DM patients who were found eligible for dual therapy (HbA1c ≥7.5%–9.0%) and were prescribed acarbose/metformin FDC as an initial therapy by treating physician. Patients of age ≥18 years who were recently diagnosed with T2DM within past 6 months were included. Study parameters were observed duringfirst visit (baseline), 6, 12 and 24 weeks as per routine practice of treating physician. Primary endpoint was mean change in HbA1c from baseline till 24 weeks.

Results: 1,714 patients from 56 centers across India were enrolled. Mean age was 49.6 ± 10.8 years. Mean HbA1c reduction from baseline (8.06 ± 0.46%) till 24 weeks (7.06 ± 0.65%) was 1% ($p < 0.0001$). 56% patients achieved HbA1c target ≤ 7%. 89.4% of patients continued the FDC without requirement of additional anti-diabetic agents for glycemic control. Mean reduction in PPG was 55.7 mg/dL and FPG was 32.0 mg/dL ($p < 0.0001$) from baseline (219.4 ± 54.1 mg/dL and 145.2 ± 35.8 mg/dL respectively) till 24 weeks. Mean weight reduction (Baseline—72.9 kg) was 2.2 kg. 97.2% patients completed the study. 0.94% experienced drug related treatment emergent adverse event (TEAE), of which the most common was GI disorder. 0.82% discontinued the treatment. No fatality was recorded. FDC was overall well-tolerated.

Conclusion: Study concludes that acarbose-metformin FDC provides significant HbA1c reduction at the end of 6 months and remarkable glycemic control as early as 6 weeks without need of any rescue therapy and therefore, can be considered as the preferred combination for initiating therapy in newly diagnosed treatment naïve T2DM patients in India who present with high starting glycemic levels and require robust durable glycemic control with minimal risk of hypoglycemia and serious events or safety concerns.

84. Diabetes and Sarcopenia

Anubha Srivastava, Jayant Agarwal

ABSTRACT

Introduction: Sarcopenia - "sarx" meaning flesh and "penia" meaning loss originates from the Greek word and was first coined by Rosenberg et al. in 1989.[1] Primary Sarcopenia affects older individuals as a result of age-related muscular atrophy. Systemic ailments that affects the overall health of muscles can lead to Secondary Sarcopenia.[2] International Classification of illness (ICD 10) has given it as code M 62.84.[3]

Diabetes and Sarcopenia are both common in Elderly. Individuals with diabetes have higher prevalence of getting sarcopenia. The occurrence rate of Sarcopenia in elderly populations varies from 9.9 to 40%, whereas among T2DM, it ranges from 15 to 44% using different diagnostic criteria.[2,4,5] The risk factors of sarcopenia are aging, malnutrition lack of physical activity, chronic condition like diabetes.

Sarcopenia is an emerging public health issue especially in elderly and diabetics and is defined as age related progressive muscle mass loss and muscle function and physical performance which results in frailty, disability, falls, fractures and hospitalisation.[6] As the older populations is expected to increase by 19.4 % by 2050 in India their seems to be rise in age-related health problems including sarcopenia. Several factors contribute to developments of sarcopenia such as sedentary life style, poor nutrition, chronic health condition such as T2DM.[5,6] Sarcopenia affects the strength and is most crucial component and an important indicator of mortality.[7]

T2DM usually contributes to sarcopenia. Impaired muscle function may contribute to sedentary lifestyle in patients with T2DM and leads to metabolic abnormalities. Hence, impaired muscle function is bidirectional leading to metabolic alterations. T2DM is a chronic metabolic disease which causes macrovascular and microvascular complications. Nowadays, Sarcopenia is considered as one of the new complications of DM and in turn lead to disability, multiple hospitalisations, fractures. Thus, it is an important issue to address and diagnose as early as possible.

Table 1 compares current definitions of sarcopenia.[1-4]

TABLE 1: Comparison of current definitions of sarcopenia.

	Low muscle strength	Low muscle mass	Poor physical performance
EWGSOP[8]	Hand grip strength: <30 kg (men) and <20 kg (women)	ALM/height^2: <7.26 kg/m^2 (men) <5.50 kg/m^2 (women) OR Skeletal muscle mass/height^2: <8.87 kg/m^2 (men) <6.42 kg/m^2 (women)	Gait speed ≤0.8 m/s (4-m course) OR SPPB score: ≤8 points
EWGSOP2[9]	Hand grip strength: <27 kg (men) and <16 kg (women) OR Chair stands time: >15s (5 rises)	ALM: 20 kg (men) and <15 kg (women) OR ALM/height^2: <7.00 kg/m^2 (men) <6.00 kg/m^2 (women)	Gait speed: ≤0.8 m/s (4-m course) OR SPPB score: ≤8 points OR TUG: ≥20 s OR 400 m walk ≥6 min or non-completion

Continued

Continued

	Low muscle strength	Low muscle mass	Poor physical performance
FNIH[10]	Hand grip strength: <26 kg (men) and <16 kg (women)	ALM/BMI: <0.789 kg/BMI (men) <0.512 kg/BMI (women)	–
IWGS[11]	–	ALM/height^2: ≤ 7.23 kg/m^2 (men) ≤ 5.67 kg/m^2 (women)	Gait speed: <1.0 m/s
AWGS[12]	Hand grip strength: <26 kg (men) and <18 kg (women)	ALM/height^2: <7.0 kg/m^2 (men) <5.4 kg/m^2 (women)	Gait speed: ≤0.8 m/s (6-m course)

(EWGSOP: European working group on sarcopenia in older people; EWGSOP2: European working group on sarcopenia in older people updated definition; FNIH: foundation for the national institutes of health biomarkers consortium sarcopenia project; IWGS: international working group on sarcopenia; AWGS: Asian working group for sarcopenia; ALM: appendicular lean mass; BMI: body mass index; SPPB: short physical performance battery; TUG: timed up and go)

Pathogenesis: There is mutual interrelationship between the T2DM and Sarcopenia. Major mechanisms by which diabetes causes sarcopenia are increased insulin resistance, advanced glycation end products, chronic inflammation and oxidative stress.[7]

Skeletal muscles are one of the target organs not only for insulin action but also for location of GLUT4 receptors which gets decline with age and chronic conditions. There also occurs fat transformation leading to diabetes. The imbalance between muscle protein anabolic and catabolic pathways in the muscles lead to impaired insulin action promotes protein degradation and hamper protein synthesis resulting in loss of muscle mass and strength. Smoking, vitamin D, physical inactivity are other contributing factors.[8]

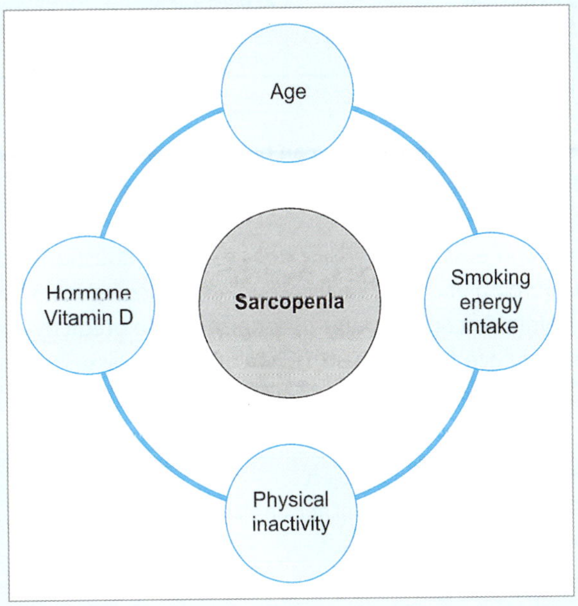

Assessment of Sarcopenia

The three dynamic approaches by measuring changes in:

1. Muscle strength (handgrip strength),
2. Physical performance (usual gait speed), and
3. Appendicular skeletal muscle mass (ASM).

TABLE 2: Comparison of various diagnostic criteria for sarcopenia and their cut-offs.[1]			
	Hand grip strength	**Muscle mass**	**Gait speed**
AWGS 2019	<28 for men <18 for women	ALM/Ht2: <7 kg/m^2—men <5.4 kg/m^2—women	<1 m/s
AGWS 2014	<26 for men <18 for women	ALM/Ht^2: <7 kg/m^2—men <5.4 kg/m^2—women	≤0.8 m/s
EWGSOP	<30 for men <20 for women	ALM/Ht^2: <7.2 kg/m^2—men <5.5 kg/m^2—women	≤0.8 m/s
EWGSOP2	<27 for men <16 for women	ALM/Ht^2: <7 kg/m^2—men <6 kg/m^2—women	≤0.8 m/s
FNIH	<26 for men <16 for women	ALM/BMI: <0.789 kg/BMI—men <0.512 kg/BMI—women	<0.8 m/s
IWGS	-	ALM/Ht^2: <7.23 kg/m^2—men <5.67 kg/m^2—women	<1 m/s
SWAG SARCO	<27.5 for men <18 for women	ALM/Ht^2: <6.11 kg/m^2—men <4.61 kg/m^2—women	≤0.8 m/s

(ALM: appendicular lean mass; BMI: body mass index)

Hence Early diagnosis and management of diabetes can help in prevention of Sarcopenia.

Some tools have been studied for assessing risk like the SARC-F questionnaire, the Red Flag method, the SMI method.

SARC-F – is one of the popular and easy test. This includes asking 5 questions addressing strength, assistance in walking, rising from a chair, stair climbing and falls. Each component is scored from 0 to 2 points, giving a global score of the SARC-F between 0 and 10 points. A score ≥ 4 points is reported to be predictive of sarcopenia and poor outcomes and could be a trigger for a more detailed assessment of sarcopenia an assessment of sarcopenia in individuals at increased risk.[9,10]

Red Flag method:[9]

Clinician's observation	• General weakness of the subject • Visual identification of loss of muscle mass • Low walking speed
General weakness of the subject	• Loss of weight • Loss of muscle strength, in arms or in legs • General weakness • Fatigue • Falls • Mobility impairment • Loss of energy • Difficulties in physical activities or activities of daily living
Clinician's assessment	• Nutrition • Body weight • Physical activity

Tests for assessment of sarcopenia: Once tests on daily screening suggests sarcopenia a detailed assessment of muscle mass using DXA or other equivalents tests can be done. The strength and muscular function can also be tested using Jamar dynamometer, or similar hydraulic dynamometer which is the gold standard. Patient is asked to squeeze for 5–6s and 6 measurements can be done. The Short physical performance battery test (SPPB) test scores maximum of 12 points which comprises of gait speed (over 3–4 m), a balance test and a repeated chair stand test focussing on lower extremity function. The SPPB is easy and takes only 10 min to complete. A score of ≤8 points have poor physical performance. The Timed Up and Go (TUG) test can be used alone for assessment by asking patients to rise from a standard armchair, walk to a marker 3 m away, turn, walk back and sit down again. The 6-min walk distance or 400 m walk time can be used to measure aerobic capacity.[9,10]

Assessment of muscle mass	Assessment of muscle strength	Assessment of physical performance
• DXA • Anthropometric measurements • CT-scan • MRI • BIA	• Handgrip strength • Lower limb muscle strength • Repeated chair stands test	• Gait speed • Timed Up and Go test • Balance test • 6-min walk test • 400 m walk test • Stair climb test • SPPB test

(SPPB: short physical performance battery; DXA: dual-energy X-ray absorptiometry; CT: computer tomography; MRI: magnetic resonance imaging; BIA: bioelectrical impedance)

MANAGEMENT

Non-Pharmacological Approaches

Physical Exercise

The most effective lifestyle intervention for the prevention of diabetes is exercise. The guidelines also recommend exercise as the main treatment for sarcopenia. Aerobic and resistance exercise both can help in preventing and treating the age related loss in muscle mass and strength. Aerobic exercise has shown to reduce the level of glucose parameters and HbA1c by improving IR, and hence, improving skeletal mass. Resistance exercise (RE) can also improve muscle strength.

Nutrition Supplementation:

Valine, leucine, and isoleucine are the branched-chain amino acids which can reduce muscle mass loss . Omega-3 fatty acids, nicotinamide adenine dinucleotide (NAD+) precursor, vitamin D and antioxidants and dietary fibres. These nutrition supplements can improve insulin sensitivity and reduce oxidative stress and inflammation which can maintain muscle mass. Beta-hydroxy-beta-methylbutyrate (HMB) in studies have shown to improve lean mass and preserve muscle strength and function in elderly and diabetics.[10]

Pharmacotherapy

There are currently no approved specific drugs for the therapy of sarcopenia.

Table 3: Effects of drug therapy on muscle and adverse side effects in diabetics medication.

Drugs	Effects on Muscle mass
Transdermal testosterone gels	Increases
Selective androgen receptor modulators (SARMs)	Increases
Metformin	Increases
Thiazolidinediones	Increases
Sulfonylureas	Decreases
Glinides	Decreases
GLP-1RA	Inconclusive
SGLT-2i	Inconclusive
Insulin	Decreases
DPPIV i	Increases

Future Prospects

Other potential therapy includes Mitochondrial-targeted antioxidants to reverse oxidative dysfunction, lower ATP levels and restore protein synthesis and muscle mass. Activin, n-terminal propeptide of procollagen III and myostatin are some biochemical markers of muscle metabolism.[10,11]

Conclusion

T2DM and sarcopenia are closely associated with one another. Muscle health impairment may contribute to progression of T2DM. Some risk factors that be contributing to sarcopenia in diabetes could be age, higher insulin resistance, chronic inflammation, high oxidative stress, accumulation of AGEs, ectopic fat accumulation, deficiency of vitamins. Management should be individualised to patients from selection of oral hypoglycaemic agents to specific exercises and protein-rich nutrition.

REFERENCES

1. Chen LK, Woo J, Chai PA, Auyeung TW, Chou MY, Iijima K, et al. Asian Working Group for Sarcopenia: 2019 Consensus Update on Sarcopenia Diagnosis and Treatment. J Am Med Dir Assoc. 2020;21:300-7.e2.
2. S Das et al; The impact of diabetes on sarcopenia in community-dwelling older adults in India: Key findings from the longitudinal ageing study in India(LASI); Diabetes Epidemiology and Management 12 (2023) 100158.
3. Newman AB, Kupelian V, Visser M, Simonsick EM, Goodpaster BH, Kritchevsky SB, et al. Strength, But Not Muscle Mass, Is Associated with Mortality in the Health, Aging and Body Composition Study Cohort. J. Gerontol. A Biol. Sci. Med. Sci. 2006;61:72-77.
4. Rosenberg IH. Sarcopenia: Origins and Clinical Relevance. J. Nutr. 1997;127:990S-991S.
5. Haase CB, Brodersen JB, Bülow J. Sarcopenia: Early prevention or overdiagnosis? BMJ. 2022;376:e052592.
6. Cao L, Morley JE. Sarcopenia Is Recognized as an Independent Condition by an International Classification of Disease, Tenth Revision, Clinical Modification (ICD-10-CM) Code. J. Am. Med. Dir. Assoc. 2016;17:675-77.
7. Cruz-Jentoft AJ, Landi F, Schneider SM, Zuniga C, Arai H, Boirie Y, et al. Prevalence of and interventions for sarcopenia in ageing adults: A systematic review. Report of the International Sarcopenia Initiative (EWGSOP and IWGS) Age Ageing. 2014;43:748-59.
8. Kaur P, Bansal R, Bhargava B, Mishra S, Gill H, Mithal A. Decreased handgrip strength in patients with type 2 diabetes: A cross-sectional study in a tertiary care hospital in north India. Diabetes Metab. Syndr. Clin. Res. Rev. 2021;15:325–329.
9. Chen et al: The Association Between Sarcopenia and Diabetes: From Pathophysiology Mechanism to Therapeutic Strategy; Diabetes, Metabolic Syndrome and Obesity 2023:16.
10. Beaudart, C., McCloskey, E., Bruyère, O. et al. Sarcopenia in daily practice: assessment and management. BMC Geriatr 16, 170 (2016).
11. Oktaviana J, Zanker J, Vogrin S, Duque G. The Effect of β-hydroxy-β-methylbutyrate (HMB) on Sarcopenia and Functional Frailty in Older Persons: A Systematic Review. J Nutr Health Aging. 2019;23(2):145-50.

85. Multimorbidity: The Future Model for Holistic Care

Kamlesh Khunti

ABSTRACT

Multimorbidity: The future model for holistic care

Multimorbidity or multiple long-term conditions, defined as the coexistence of two or more chronic conditions, is increasingly prevalent among individuals with type 2 diabetes mellitus (T2DM). Multimorbidity is associated with increased healthcare utilisation, polypharmacy, and a heightened risk of adverse outcomes, including reduced quality of life and increased mortality. This complexity poses significant challenges for conventional care models that often focus on single-disease management. Conditions commonly co-occurring with T2DM, such as cardiovascular disease, chronic kidney disease, and mental health disorders, interact in complex ways, often amplifying disease burden and complicating treatment strategies. Traditional siloed care models fail to address these interactions and may exacerbate fragmentation in care delivery. A future model for holistic care emphasises integrated, multidisciplinary approaches that prioritise the patient's overall health, preferences, and goals. Key components include tailored treatment regimens, shared decision-making, and coordinated care across specialties. Embracing technology, such as telemedicine and health informatics, further enhances patient engagement and care continuity. A holistic approach to care is needed to address the unique needs of this population and improve clinical outcomes. By integrating multidisciplinary teams, leveraging technology, and addressing systemic barriers, these models align with the complex needs of individuals with T2DM and multimorbidity.

Are current strategies delivering holistic treatment approach for people with living with T2 diabetes?

Type 2 diabetes mellitus (T2DM) is a complex, multifaceted condition requiring a holistic approach that addresses glycaemic control, comorbidities, and psychosocial well-being. Despite advancements in treatment strategies, current care delivery often falls short of meeting these comprehensive needs. Current approaches to T2DM management remain largely focused on achieving glycaemic targets through pharmacotherapy, lifestyle interventions, and regular monitoring. Despite the evidence base, these strategies have failed to improve disease outcomes at population levels. Fragmented care models fail to address the interplay between diabetes and its comorbidities, such as cardiovascular disease, mental health disorders, and obesity. Other critical barriers to optimal care is therapeutic inertia—the delay in initiating or intensifying treatment despite unmet clinical goals as well as poor adherence in routine clinical practice. Interventions to improve outcomes include multidisciplinary models of care, methods to overcome therapeutic inertia and improve adherence to medications improve risk factor control as well as structured education programmes.

Importance of early glycaemic control

Early glycaemic control in type 2 diabetes mellitus (T2DM) is increasingly recognised as a cornerstone of effective diabetes management. Achieving and maintaining near-normal glycaemic levels early in the course of T2DM significantly reduces the risk of both microvascular and macrovascular complications. Evidence from landmark studies, such as the UKPDS (United Kingdom Prospective Diabetes Study), demonstrates that intensive glycaemic control reduces the incidence of retinopathy, nephropathy, and neuropathy. Furthermore, a "legacy effect" or "metabolic memory" of early glycaemic control underscores its long-term cardiovascular benefits, even when subsequent glycaemic levels fluctuate. Early intervention also slows β-cell dysfunction and insulin resistance progression, preserving endogenous insulin secretion and potentially altering the disease trajectory.

Lifestyle modifications initiated alongside pharmacological interventions lead to benefits of early control. Additionally, early glycaemic control positively impacts psychological well-being by mitigating the burden of complications and enhancing patient confidence in disease self-management. Despite advancements in pharmacological and lifestyle interventions, suboptimal glycaemic control in the early stages of the disease remains prevalent, leading to progressive complications.

86. Can Cardiovascular Risk Reduction be the Sole Criterion for Selection of Diabetes Drugs

Akashkumar N Singh

ABSTRACT

Diabetes is a growing global health concern, significantly associated with cardiovascular disease, which is a leading cause of morbidity and mortality in diabetic individuals.

Indian studies like ICMR-INDIAB-17, a study by Unnikrishnan et al., and CINDI-2 have reported a high prevalence of diabetes and associated cardiovascular risk factors in urban and rural populations, even in younger diabetics.

Insulin resistance and metabolic syndrome contribute to the high burden of cardiovascular diseases in prediabetes and diabetes. The overproduction of free radicals and the resulting oxidative stress leads to endothelial dysfunction, a precursor to atherosclerosis and is an early indicator of cardiovascular disease. Inflammatory factors also play a critical role in the development and progression of atherothrombosis and plaque rupture. Antidiabetic medications that exhibit anti-inflammatory and anti-atherogenic properties, such as thiazolidinediones and GLP-1 receptor agonists, may offer additional benefits beyond glycaemic control in reducing cardiovascular risk.

Major studies done did not consistently show benefits of Intense glucose control in terms of macrovascular disease prevention in patients of T2D. However, the advent of newer antidiabetic agents, such as sodium-glucose cotransporter-2 inhibitors (SGLT2i) and glucagon-like peptide-1 receptor agonists (GLP-1 RAs), has led to a paradigm shift in the management of cardiovascular risk in patients with T2D. These therapies have demonstrated significant reductions in the risk of major adverse cardiovascular events, hospitalisation for heart failure, and cardiovascular, renal and all-cause mortality in large-scale clinical trials.

Furthermore, the SGLT2 inhibitors have shown promising results in improving cardiovascular outcomes in patients with diabetes and kidney disease.

Therefore, considering the elevated cardiovascular risk profile of diabetic patients, there is a need to prioritise therapies with demonstrated cardiovascular risk reduction benefits in addition to their glucose-lowering capabilities.

The guidelines for the management of type 2 diabetes now emphasise the importance of considering cardiovascular risk reduction when selecting antidiabetic medications.

Cardiovascular risk reduction should be a key consideration in the selection of antidiabetic medications for patients with type 2 diabetes. The availability of therapies with proven cardiovascular and renal benefits, such as SGLT2 inhibitors and GLP-1 receptor agonists, has transformed the approach to diabetes management.

87. Topic Liraglutide Biosimilar The Game Changer for Managing Diabesity in India

Ameya Joshi

ABSTRACT

Type 2 diabetes mellitus (T2DM) is in epidemic proportions in India and the main characteristic of Indian T2DM is obesity which can be visceral or overall (based on body mass index). As a result, there is a high prevalence of T2DM with cardiovascular disease in India. As per guidelines the GLP1 receptor agonists (GLP-1RA) have been the standard of care for these people with T2DM. Liraglutide is one of the oldest GLP1RA available in the Indian market initially marketed as VICTOZA by novo nordisk. Liraglutide helps in effectively controlling blood glucose levels in addition to aiding weight loss. It has also proven to be cardioprotective. However, it remained underpenetrated among large deserving populations due to the price. Introducing biosimilars of liraglutide represents a significant advancement in diabetes management in India. This affordable alternative has been supported by robust clinical evidence showing its efficacy in managing T2DM alongside atherosclerotic cardiovascular diseases (ASCVD) and obesity. Clinical trials have revealed comparable safety and efficacy profiles of biosimilar to the reference product, confirming its effectiveness in achieving glycemic control and potentially improving cardiac and renal safety outcomes among patients. The availability of liraglutide biosimilars in India can improve treatment adherence and patient outcomes, particularly in the context of an increasing number of individuals seeking effective weight loss and diabetes management options. As the prevalence of diabetes continues to rise in India, the accessibility of liraglutide biosimilars provides a critical resource for healthcare professionals and patients alike, enhancing the landscape of diabetes care and management in the region.

88. Bone and Diabetes

Vivien Lim

ABSTRACT

Diabetes is a metabolic disorder characterized by high blood glucose levels, which can lead to myriad complications affecting various organs and systems, including bone health. There is a cross talk and linkage between diabetes and bone such that patients with diabetes have higher risk of osteoporosis and fractures. This association occurs for both Type 1 and Type 2 diabetes though the reasons underlining this increased risk might not be fully similar. The T-score per se might also underestimate the fracture risk for this group of patients. At the same time, some diabetic drugs and common drugs that a patient with diabetes might be prescribed might worsen the issue.

The talk will aim to provide an overview of the following:

- Relationship between diabetes and bone touching on mechanisms of impact on the bone
- The clinical implications in patients with diabetes, including increased risk of osteoporosis with increased fracture risk at a higher T-score level.
- Approach to bone health in patients with diabetes:
    - Interpretation of the bone mineral density in these patients
    - Glucose control including medication choice
    - Lifestyle modification

89. Use of BMI in DCES Practice Give it Up

Balaji Jaganmohan

ABSTRACT

The Body Mass Index (BMI), a tool traditionally used to classify body weight relative to height, has faced growing scrutiny for its inadequacy in modern diabetes care and education specialist (DCES) practices. Recent evidence underscores its limitations in capturing the complexity of health and diabetes management, necessitating a transition to more holistic and individualized measures.

BMI simplifies health assessment by failing to differentiate between muscle mass and fat mass, often resulting in misleading classifications. It also does not distinguish between metabolically harmful visceral fat and less harmful subcutaneous fat—a critical factor in diabetes risk evaluation. Furthermore, BMI ignores essential individual differences such as age, gender, ethnicity, and genetics, which significantly impact diabetes outcomes. Its neglect of fat distribution, a key indicator of metabolic health, further highlights its insufficiency.[1,4]

As a metric for tracking progress, BMI is flawed. It does not reflect improvements in metabolic health from lifestyle changes, such as reduced visceral fat or enhanced insulin sensitivity. For instance, increases in muscle mass may elevate BMI despite substantial health benefits. Moreover, reliance on BMI perpetuates weight stigma and risks misdiagnosis, stigmatizing individuals based on weight while overlooking those with unhealthy fat distributions but lower BMI values.[2,5]

Alternative measures provide a more nuanced understanding of diabetes risk and health progress. Waist-to-hip ratio, body fat percentage, and waist circumference better capture fat distribution and metabolic health. Advanced tools, such as continuous glucose monitoring (CGM), offer actionable insights that align with individualized care.[3] Replacing BMI with these evidence-based practices empowers DCES professionals to address root causes of poor health, including nutrition, stress, sleep, and physical activity, fostering sustainable, patient-centered behavior changes.

This shift from BMI to more meaningful health metrics aligns with the evolving needs of diabetes care, emphasizing holistic, evidence-driven approaches to improve patient outcomes and overall well-being.

REFERENCES

1. Kramer, H, et al. "Identifying Preferred Features of Weight Loss Programs for Adults with Type 2 Diabetes." Diabetes Care, vol. 47, no. 4, 2024, pp. 739-748. https://diabetesjournals.org/care/article/47/4/739/154274/Identifying-Preferred-Features-of-Weight-Loss
2. Prentice, AM, and Jebb, SA. "Beyond Body Mass Index." Obesity Reviews, vol. 2, no. 3, 2001, pp. 141-147. https://pmc.ncbi.nlm.nih.gov/articles/PMC11204233/
3. Gutin, B. "Inadequacy of BMI for Studies of Body Fatness and Health Risks." Current Opinion in Clinical Nutrition and Metabolic Care, vol. 14, no. 6, 2011, pp. 523-527. https://pmc.ncbi.nlm.nih.gov/articles/PMC2930234/
4. "Use and Misuse of BMI Categories." AMA Journal of Ethics, July 2023. https://journalofethics.ama-assn.org/article/use-and-misuse-bmi-categories/2023-07
5. "BMI a Poor Metric for Measuring People's Health, Say Experts." Harvard T.H. Chan School of Public Health, 2023. https://hsph.harvard.edu/news/bmi-a-poor-metric-for-measuring-peoples-health-say-experts/

90. GLP1RA—Beyond Glycemic Control

Mohammed Yousuf Khan

ABSTRACT

All the international guidelines recommend GLP1 receptor agonists (GLP1RA) as the first line agents for type 2 diabetics with ASCVD. The role of GLP1RA in Diabetes management is just the tip of the iceberg, as they have potential role to play in almost all organ systems of the human body.

GLP 1 receptor (GLP-1R) belongs to the GPCR (G protein coupled receptor) family and is expressed on the surfaces of various tissue cells in the human body, apart from pancreas. GLP-1R has multiple biological effects, such as improving cardiovascular function, reducing neuroinflammation, promoting nerve growth, suppressing appetite and causing satiety, delaying gastric emptying, regulating blood lipid metabolism and reducing fat deposition, improving MASLD (metabolic dysfunction associated steatotic liver disease). There is growing data and evidence for GLP-1RAs in treating musculoskeletal disorders, neurodegenerative diseases, and various carcinomas. For example, in the treatment of Alzheimer's diseases (AD) and Parkinson's disease (PD), GLP-1RAs have shown potential in slowing the disease progression, while their anti-inflammatory properties offer new hope for conditions such as osteoarthritis (OA), rheumatoid arthritis (RA) and Psoriasis.

For example, in fibroblast-like RA synoviocytes, the administration of lixisenatide resulted in a reduction in the inflammatory response. This was achieved by decreasing the expression of proinflammatory cytokines such as tumor necrosis factor (TNF), interleukin-6 (IL-6), and interleukin-8.

GLP-1RAs are also showing promising results in enhancing Exercise Endurance. These Studies indicate that acute exercise and short-term endurance training significantly increase GLP-1 secretion in mice. In endurance-trained men, GLP-1 plasma concentrations are elevated immediately at 30 and 45 minutes after exercise.

In the field of obesity, GLP1RA have become the show stoppers. Starting with exenatide, followed by liraglutide and Dulaglutide, now the newer Semaglutide is a single receptor GLP1RA providing upto 8% weight loss, while dual receptor GLP1RA Terzepatide and triple receptor GLP1RA Ritatrutide have potential for 15% and 20% weight loss respectively. Orforglipron and Danuglipron are the oral GLP-1RA in the pipeline.

The future of GLP-1RA therapy is promising with more efficient formulations, such as long-acting and oral versions, to improve patient compliance. With increasing clinical evidence, GLP-1RAs are set to become essential in treating complex and chronic diseases.

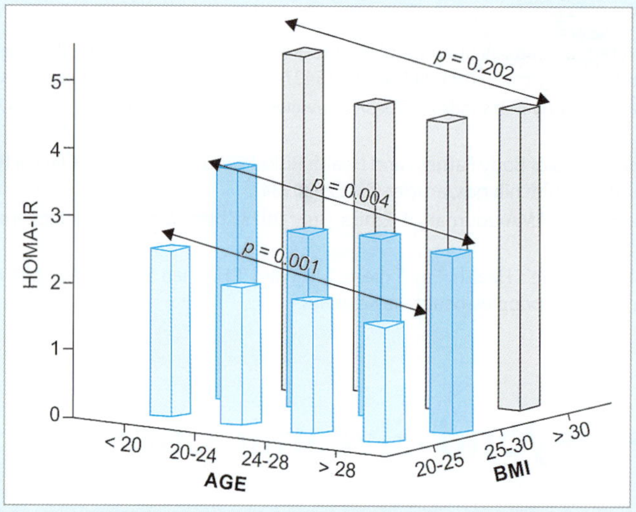

The gradual improvement of insulin resistance over the years in normal weight (light cyan bars) and over weight (cyan bars) women with polycystic ovary syndrome, but not in their obese counterparts (gray bars).

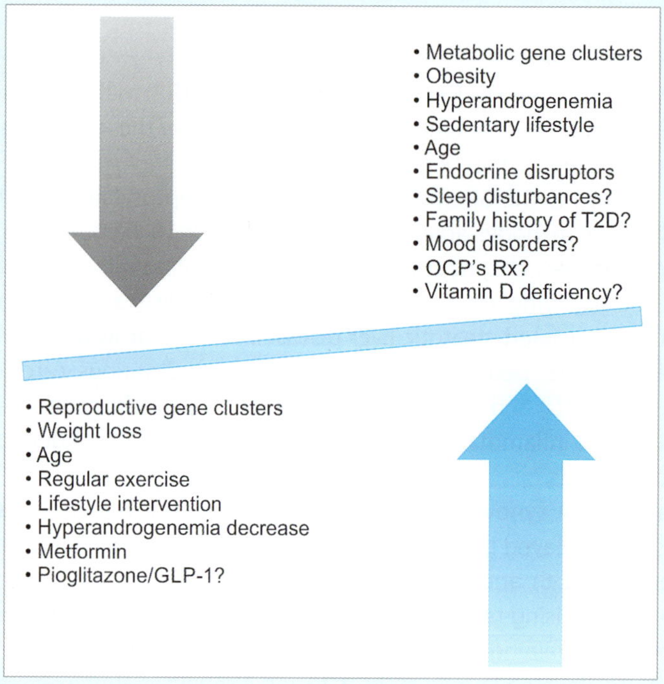

The interaction of positive (cyan arrow) and negative (gray arrow) factors affecting dysglycemia in women with polycystic ovary syndrome.

TABLE 1: Guidelines regarding oral glucose tolerance test upon diagnosis of Polycystic ovary syndrome.

Ref.	OGTT recommended upon diagnosis in all women with PCOS	Follow-up with OGTT
Joint AACE/ACE and AE-PCOS society	Yes	(1) Yearly in woment with IGT; and (2) Every 1–2 years based on BMI (not specified) and family history of T2D
Australian NHMRC	Recommended if one or more criteria exist: (1) BMI > 25 kg/m^2 or in Asians > 23 kg/m^2; (2) History of IFG, IGT, GDM; (3) Family history of T2D; (4) Arterial hypertension; and (5) High-risk ethnicity	Every 1–3 years, based on presence of other diabetes risk factors
Endocrine Society	Yes	Every 3–5 years (Sooner if additional risk factors for T2D develop)
Royal College of Obstetricians and Gynecology	Recommended if one or more criteria exist: (1) BMI ≥ 25 kg/m^2 (2) Age ≥ 40 years; (3) Previous GDM; and (4) Family history of T2D	Yearly in woment with IGT or IFG
AE-PCOS Society	Recommended if one or more criteria exist: (1) BMI ≥ 30 kg/m^2 (2) Age ≥ 40 years; (3) Previous GDM; and (4) Family history of T2D	Every 2 years in women with risk factors (Sooner if additional risk factors for T2D develop)
ESHRE and ASRM	Recommended if BMI ≥ 27 kg/m^2	Not specified

(OGTT: oral glucose tolerance test; PCOS: polycystic ovary syndrome; T2D: type 2 diabetes mellitus; BMI: body mass index; IFG: impaired fasting glucose; IGT: impaired glucose tolerance)

91. Reducing Microvascular Risk in Diabetes—Insight from Recent Trials

Michel P Hermans

ABSTRACT

Beyond key landmark prospective trials on glycemic control and non-ophtalmological interventions on diabetic retinopathy (DRP) in type 1 (T1D) and type 2 diabetes (T2D), the ACCORD Glycaemic control (T2D) and other fenofibrate trials such as FIELD (T2D), ACCORD-Eye (T2D), and a recent Korean registry (T2D), as well as the LENS study (T2D and T1D), suggest microvascular benefit despite neutral effects of PPAR-α agonism on ASCVD outcomes. In a large RWE propensity-matched cohort registry, addition of fenofibrate to statins was associated with risk reduction of the primary outcome (a DRP progression composite) in T2D patients with MetS and baseline DRP, without interaction between patients characteristics and treatment benefit. In LENS (Lowering Events in Non-proliferative Retinopathy in Scotland), fenofibrate versus placebo reduced DRP progression by 27% in diabetic patients with early DRP at baseline. The incidence of macular oedema was also markedly lowered by fenofibrate. LENS extends the evidence for a benefit of fenofibrate on DRP, hitherto only studied in T2D, to T1D patients, since the T1D subgroup on fenofibrate (>25% of the cohort) profited as much as T2D patients. This points to non-lipid mechanisms underlying the effect of PPAR-α agonism on DRP, since atherogenic dyslipidemia is uncommon in T1D.

REFERENCES

1. Hiukka A, Maranghi M, Matikainen N, Taskinen MR. PPARalpha: an emerging therapeutic target in diabetic microvascular damage. Nat Rev Endocrinol. 2010;6(8):454-63.
2. Nam Hoon Kim, Jimi Choi, Young Ho Kim, Hwa Lee, Sin Gon Kim. Addition of fenofibrate to statins is associated with risk reduction of diabetic retinopathy progression in patients with type 2 diabetes and metabolic syndrome: A propensity-matched cohort study. Diabetes Metab. 2023;49(3):101428.
3. Preiss D, Logue J, Sammons E, Zayed M, Emberson J, Wade R, et al. Effect of fFenofibrate on progression of diabetic retinopathy. NEJM Evid. 2024;3:EVIDoa2400179.
4. Varughese MS, Nayak AU, Jacob S. Fenofibrate therapy in reducing the progression of diabetic retinopathy: revisiting the FIELD and ACCORD-EYE studies through the LENS trial. Eye (Lond). 2025;39(1):15-7.

92. Paediatric Diabetes Symposium

László Barkai

ABSTRACT

Damage to the peripheral nervous system is a well-known complication of diabetes, however, the involvement of the central nervous system is a less explored phenomenon. In recent years, special attention has been paid to childhood-onset type 1 diabetes (T1D), as the effects on the developing nervous system can cause both structural and functional abnormalities. In children and adolescents with T1D, neuro-cognitive examination methods have shown alterations in memory, learning, task execution skills, among others. Recent studies pointed out to attention deficits, however, in the case of some psychic manifestations, familial aggregation could also be detected. With the help of modern imaging techniques, pathological phenomena in the morphology and volume of white and gray matter, the growth rate of the brain tissue, the lesions of the temporal lobe and cuneus area were revealed. In addition to these, neurochemical studies have also documented shifts in the levels of certain neurotransmitters. Previous studies have emphasized the role of recurrent hypoglycaemias in the background of these phenomena. However, subsequent studies have shown that the pathological role of chronic hyperglycaemia could be even more significant etiological factor. In addition, very young onset of T1D and presentation ketoacidosis have proven to be additional risk factors. The literature also points out that subtile cognitive dysfunction due to mild brain damage as a result of poor metabolic control can also negatively affect the success of long-term care, impairing the therapy adherence and self-management of patients with T1D. However, based on preliminary studies, it appears that adverse effects on the developing central nervous system may be preventable or reversible with meticulous glycaemic control.

93. Insulin Therapy in Pregnancy: Balancing Maternal Health and Foetal Outcomes

Lotika Purohit

ABSTRACT

In order to manage gestational diabetes mellitus (GDM) and pre-existing diabetes and provide the best possible health outcomes for both the mother and the foetus, insulin therapy throughout pregnancy is essential. To reduce hazards for the woman and her growing foetus, proper glucose control is crucial. While maternal hypoglycaemia carries its own hazards, uncontrolled hyperglycaemia can result in complications like preeclampsia, macrosomia, and an increased chance of caesarean birth. Throughout pregnancy, insulin medication must be closely monitored and adjusted to provide strict glucose control without causing hypoglycaemia.

Each person's needs determine which insulin therapy is best for them, including whether to utilize long-acting, rapid-acting, or insulin pumps. Insulin should be used as the first line of treatment when diet and lifestyle changes are not enough, according to current data.

Optimizing foetal growth, avoiding excessive weight gain, and maintaining maternal health are the objectives. However, as changes in the mother's blood glucose can have a direct impact on the development of the foetus and may result in negative outcomes such birth abnormalities, stillbirth, and neonatal hypoglycaemia, the effect of insulin therapy on foetal outcomes needs to be properly monitored.

Comprehensive prenatal care involves not only insulin but also frequent blood glucose monitoring, dietary modifications, and physical activity. To achieve the delicate balance needed for both mother well-being and favourable foetal outcomes, obstetricians, diabetologists, and dietitians must work together. With an emphasis on maximizing the health of both the mother and the foetus through individualized treatment approaches, this review addresses the advantages, difficulties, and best practices of managing insulin medication throughout pregnancy.

94. Brief Update on MASH; Implications for Diabetes

Rita Basu

ABSTRACT

Metabolic dysfunction-associated steatotic liver disease (MASLD) and metabolic dysfunction-associated steatohepatitis (MASH), has recently had a change in nomenclature from NAFLD and NASH respectively. Globally, the prevalence of MAFLD is 25%, with 12–14% of those cases progressing to the more severe form, MASH. The highest rates of MAFLD and MASH are found in Middle Eastern countries, and prevalence is notably higher in individuals with type 2 diabetes (T2D) and visceral obesity. Among those with obesity, 25–30% have MASH, and 30–40% of people with diabetes are affected. The prevalence of MAFLD is expected to rise, with an increasing number of individuals developing advanced forms of the disease. Estimates suggest that 20% of people with MASH could develop serious liver complications, including cirrhosis, and MASH has become a leading cause of hepatocellular carcinoma (HCC). This growing trend is particularly concerning for regions such as Asia and the Middle East. Until recently, there were no specific treatments for MASH. However, the US FDA has conditionally approved resmetirom for treating moderate to advanced MASH, specifically for patients with fibrosis stages 2 or 3. There are currently no FDA-approved noninvasive tests to diagnose metabolic dysfunction-associated steatohepatitis (MASH) with fibrosis stages F2–F3 or to monitor treatment response. Guidelines from the American Association for the Study of Liver Diseases (AASLD) emphasize the limitations of liver biopsy, leading to the use of noninvasive liver disease assessment (NILDA) tests. Among these, imaging-based NILDAs, such as liver stiffness measurement (LSM) through vibration-controlled transient elastography (VCTE) or magnetic resonance elastography (MRE), provide better accuracy for assessing fibrosis than blood-based tests. Other medications including GLP-1 RA, Dual and triple agonists as well as aggressive management of obesity and metabolic dysfunction are cornerstone of management of this condition in people with diabetes.

95. How to Prescribe Exercise in Those with Sarcopenia, Obesity, and Diabetes

Mikel Izquierdo

ABSTRACT

With the global population aging, a critical question emerges: how can we enhance older adults' quality of life while minimizing age-related diseases and disabilities? Evidence supports exercise as both preventive and therapeutic, playing a pivotal role in extending healthy longevity, preventing chronic conditions, and preserving physical and cognitive function. The "Global Consensus on Optimal Exercise Recommendations for Enhancing Healthy Longevity in Older Adults (ICFSR)" underscores the importance of tailored exercise programs in geriatric care, positioning exercise as a key intervention against age-related decline.[1]

Exercise is particularly effective in slowing disuse syndromes and improving outcomes in conditions such as Parkinson's disease, chronic obstructive pulmonary disease, and cardiometabolic disorders.[2] However, addressing glycemic control without tackling central obesity and sedentary lifestyles can worsen complications and increase polypharmacy in individuals with insulin resistance. Diet-induced weight loss alone can result in lean tissue loss, aggravating sarcopenia and osteopenia.[1]

Consensus guidelines recommend 3–4 hours per week of moderate-to-high-intensity aerobic exercise to improve insulin sensitivity, manage weight, and reduce cardiovascular risks in individuals with type 2 diabetes (T2D).[1,3] However, comorbidities such as cognitive decline, osteoarthritis, ischemic heart disease, and hypertension can limit adherence to these recommendations, making high-volume aerobic exercise unrealistic for many older adults.

Progressive Resistance Training (PRT) presents an alternative approach for older adults with T2D, improving muscle and bone mass, glucose uptake, visceral fat reduction, and functional status while enhancing sleep and modo.[1] Unlike aerobic exercise, PRT specifically combats sarcopenia, which is essential for preventing dementia, though more research is needed.

In frail older adults with diabetes, a combined approach involving PRT, nutritional education, and adjusted clinical targets for blood glucose and blood pressure has demonstrated functional benefits(4). Multicomponent programs that include resistance, endurance, balance, and gait training can enhance functional capacity, reduce falls, and delay institutionalization and disability.[1,4]

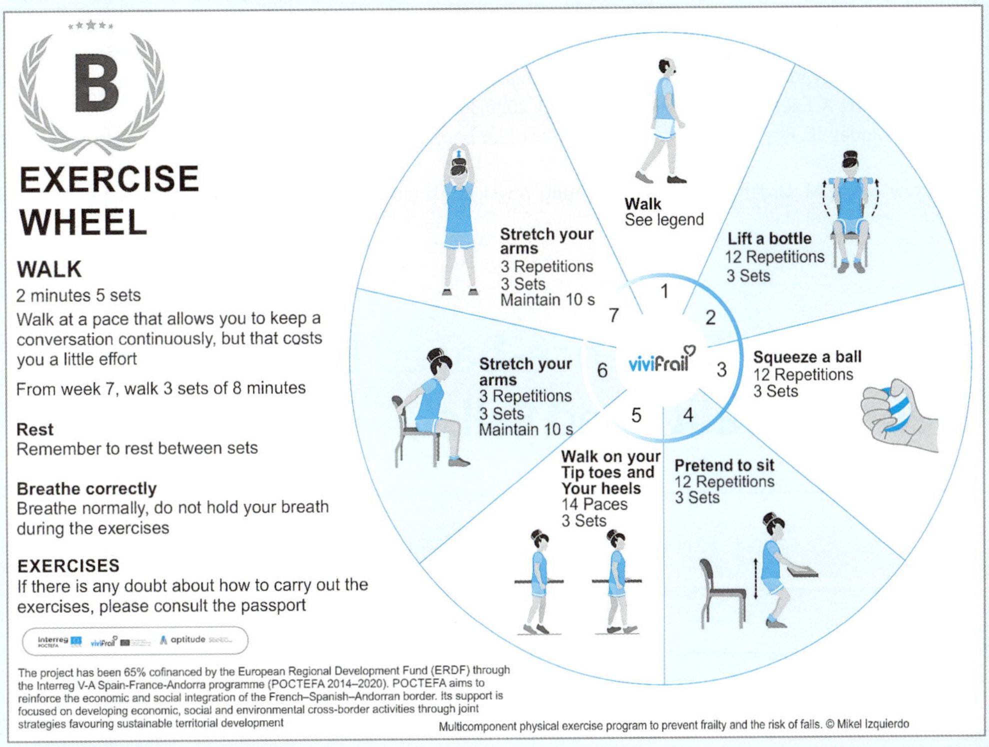

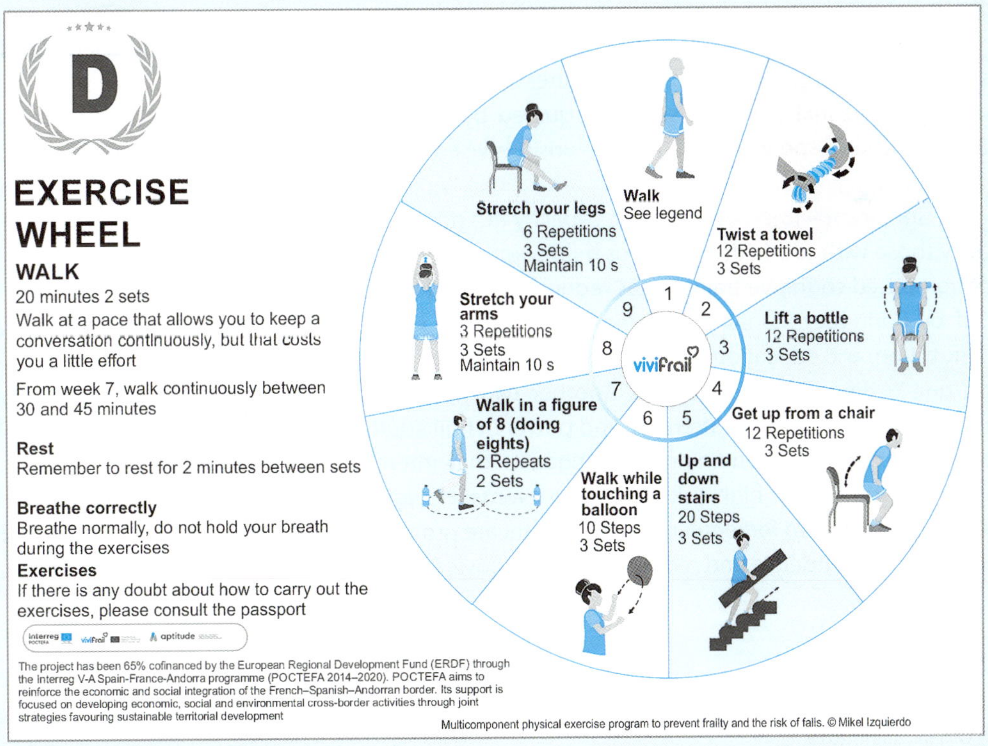

Figure 1: Exercise wheel type B (frail) is for older people who can walk with difficulty or help (1), and type D (robust) is for a person who has minimal physical limitations or no limitations (2). Retrieved from (Izquierdo M, et al. Multicomponent Physical Exercise program VIVIFRAIL. 2019. (Multicomponent physical exercise program to prevent frailty and the risk of falls. © Mikel Izquierdo) (2)

REFERENCES

1. Izquierdo M, de Souto Barreto P, Arai H, Bischoff-Ferrari HA, Cadore EL, Cesari M, et al. Global consensus on optimal exercise recommendations for enhancing healthy longevity in older adults (ICFSR). The journal of nutrition, health & aging. 2024:100401.
2. Izquierdo M, Morley JE, Lucia A. Exercise in people over 85. BMJ. 2020;368:m402.
3. Izquierdo M, Duque G, Morley JE. Physical activity guidelines for older people: knowledge gaps and future directions. Lancet Healthy Longev. 2021;2(6):e380-e3.
4. Izquierdo M, Fiatarone Singh M. Urgent need for integrating physical exercise into geriatric medicine: a call to action. Br J Sports Med. 2023;57(15):953-4.

96. VIVIFRAIL: An Evidence-based Program for Preventing Frailty and Falls

Mikel Izquierdo

ABSTRACT

The VIVIFRAIL multicomponent physical exercise program, recommended by the WHO's ICOPE guidance, aims to prevent frailty and falls in older adults through a person-centered approach in primary care.[1] The VIVIFRAIL physical exercise guide (available at http://vivifrail.com/resources/) includes lower-limb exercises (e.g., chair squats, leg presses), upper-body exercises (e.g., seated bench press), and balance and gait retraining (e.g., single-leg standing, tandem walking, obstacle navigation). Additionally, it features proprioceptive exercises on unstable surfaces and weight transfer movements. Personalized exercise plans, guided by assessments such as the Short Physical Performance Battery (SPPB) and walking speed tests, allow for unsupervised sessions tailored to individual functional capacities (www.vivifrail.com).[2]

VIVIFRAIL has significantly improved intrinsic capacity (IC) domains like locomotion, cognition, and vitality in older adults, especially those with pre-frailty, frailty, or mild cognitive impairment.[3] Furthermore, combining VIVIFRAIL with executive function-based cognitive training has reduced falls and related adverse outcomes.

A study led by Rodriguez-Mañas et al.[4] demonstrated that incorporating VIVIFRAIL and progressive resistance training (PRT), nutrition, and education into a multimodal intervention resulted in a €420 per patient annual healthcare cost reduction due to fewer hospitalizations. Another two-year longitudinal study[4,5] found that 16 weeks of PRT improved functional capacity, muscle strength, and power in frail adults over 70 with type 2 diabetes (T2D), with some benefits persisting 38 weeks post-training. This suggests that intermittent multimodal interventions can maintain improvements in older adults at high risk of adverse events. However, insulin sensitivity benefits from exercise are short-lived, reinforcing the need for regular activity. Healthcare professionals and policymakers should promote regular exercise to preserve independence and reduce healthcare costs in older adults.

REFERENCES

1. Organization. WH. Integrated care for older people (ICOPE): guidance for person-centred assessment and pathways in primary care. Geneva: World Health Organization; 2019.
2. Izquierdo M. Multicomponent physical exercise program VIVIFRAIL 2019 [updated April 23]. Available from: https://vivifrail.com/resources/.
3. Casas-Herrero Á, Sáez de Asteasu ML, Antón-Rodrigo I, Sánchez-Sánchez JL, Montero-Odasso M, Marín-Epelde I, et al. Effects of Vivifrail multicomponent intervention on functional capacity: a multicentre, randomized controlled trial. J Cachexia Sarcopenia Muscle. 2022;13(2): 884-93.

4. Rodriguez-Manas L, Laosa O, Vellas B, Paolisso G, Topinkova E, Oliva-Moreno J, et al. Effectiveness of a multimodal intervention in functionally impaired older people with type 2 diabetes mellitus. J Cachexia Sarcopenia Muscle. 2019;10(4):721-33.
5. Izquierdo M, Laosa O, Cadore EL, Abizanda P, Garcia-Garcia FJ, Hornillos M, et al. Two-Year Follow-up of a Multimodal Intervention on Functional Capacity and Muscle Power in Frail Patients With Type 2 Diabetes. Journal of the American Medical Directors Association. 2021;22(9):1906-11.

97. Euglycemic Diabetic Ketoacidosis (eDKA): A Critical Must-Know in Modern Diabetes Care

NK Singh

ABSTRACT

Euglycemic diabetic ketoacidosis (eDKA) is a rare but life-threatening condition characterized by ketoacidosis with blood glucose levels <200 mg/dL, often leading to delayed diagnosis and treatment. It poses a significant diagnostic challenge due to normoglycemia, resulting in potentially worse outcomes compared to classic diabetic ketoacidosis (DKA). The mortality rate of typical DKA ranges from 0.65 to 3.3%, but eDKA, particularly in pregnant women, has been associated with increased maternal mortality and fetal demise (up to 9%).

The use of sodium-glucose cotransporter-2 inhibitors (SGLT-2i) has emerged as a common precipitant of eDKA, often triggered by stress, infections, surgery, or insulin dose reduction. The pathophysiology of eDKA mirrors that of DKA but involves SGLT-2i-induced glycosuria, which lowers plasma glucose while promoting ketogenesis. Early symptoms such as malaise, nausea, and mild discomfort may mask the condition, delaying critical interventions.

Diagnosis

To make a diagnosis of DKA a triad of hyperglycemia above 250 mg/dL, ketonemia, and metabolic acidosis with elevated anion gap is required

EDKA is like DKA but lacks the classic hyperglycemia component

In EDKA, blood glucose (BG) is generally <200 mg/dL, although in some reports a cut-off of 300 mg/dL has been used to define EDKA

Prefer to use a BG threshold of <200 mg/dL, ketonemia (serum β-hydroxybutyrate ≥3.0 mmol/L), and at least one of the following criteria to define EDKA:
1. Arterial pH ≤7.3
2. Serum bicarbonate ≤18 mEq/L
3. Anion gap >10

Key management strategies include early detection through serum or urine ketone testing regardless of glucose levels. Treatment involves volume expansion with crystalloids, dextrose (5–10%), and insulin infusion (0.05–0.1 U/kg/hour) until acidosis resolves. Insulin therapy should not be withheld due to normal glucose levels. SGLT-2 inhibitors should be discontinued upon diagnosis, and restarting them post-recovery should be carefully personalized to mitigate recurrence risk.

Pitfalls in management include insufficient insulin dosing, inadequate dextrose supplementation, and reliance on hydration alone. Prompt recognition and treatment typically result in good outcomes, but delays can lead to severe complications, including prolonged hospitalization, hypovolemic shock, respiratory failure, and rarely, death.

eDKA requires heightened awareness among physicians to ensure timely diagnosis, effective treatment, and patient education, particularly for high-risk groups such as pregnant women and individuals on SGLT-2i therapy.

REFERENCES

1. Seidu S, Alabraba V, Davies S, et al. SGLT2 Inhibitors – The New Standard of Care for Cardiovascular, Renal and Metabolic Protection in Type 2 Diabetes: A Narrative Review. Diabetes Ther. 2024;15(5):1099-1124.
2. Edwin Jarvis PR. Euglycemic diabetic ketoacidosis: a potential pitfall for the emergency physician. Clin Exp Emerg Med. 2023;10(1):110-3.

98. Non-Proteinuric Kidney Disease: A Silent Epidemic in Diabetes

Vipul Chavda

ABSTRACT

Non-Proteinuric diabetic kidney disease (NP-DKD) is an emerging phenotype of diabetic kidney disease (DKD) characterized by reduced renal function without significant albuminuria. Unlike the classical Proteinuric form of DKD, NP-DKD progresses silently, often going undetected until advanced stages. Epidemiological studies suggest that NP-DKD accounts for up to 40% of CKD cases in individuals with type 2 diabetes. This condition is commonly associated with microvascular ischemia, interstitial fibrosis, and tubular atrophy, rather than the glomerular injury typically seen in Proteinuric DKD.

The pathophysiology of NP-DKD involves complex mechanisms, including vascular injury, oxidative stress, and inflammation, which may occur independently of proteinuria. Risk factors include long-standing diabetes, hypertension, obesity, and aging. Diagnosis relies heavily on regular monitoring of estimated glomerular filtration rate (eGFR) since the absence of significant proteinuria may delay recognition.

Management of NP-DKD emphasizes tight control of blood glucose and blood pressure. Renin-angiotensin system blockers remain foundational, while newer therapeutic options, such as SGLT-2 inhibitors and GLP-1 receptor agonists, have shown significant benefits in reducing CKD progression and cardiovascular risk. Finerenone, a non-steroidal mineralocorticoid receptor antagonist, offers additional renal and anti-inflammatory benefits. Lifestyle modifications, including dietary interventions and exercise, play a critical role in preventing disease progression.

NP-DKD poses unique challenges for clinicians due to its silent nature and high cardiovascular morbidity. Increased awareness and proactive screening among healthcare providers are essential for timely intervention. Future research should focus on identifying biomarkers and exploring precision medicine approaches to improve outcomes in NP-DKD. Addressing this silent epidemic requires a multidisciplinary approach and patient-centric care to mitigate its growing burden.

REFERENCES

1. Alicic RZ, Rooney MT, Tuttle KR. Diabetic kidney disease: challenges, progress, and possibilities. Clin J Am Soc Nephrol. 2017;12(12):2032-45.
2. Thomas MC, Brownlee M, Susztak K, et al. Diabetic kidney disease. Nat Rev Dis Primers. 2015;1:15018.
3. Heerspink HJL, Stefánsson BV, Correa-Rotter R, et al. Dapagliflozin in patients with chronic kidney disease. N Engl J Med. 2020;383(15):1436-46.

99. Cognitive Decline and Diabetes: A Vicious Cycle

Veer Bahadur Singh

ABSTRACT

Both type 1 (T1DM) and type 2 diabetes mellitus (T2DM) have been associated with reduced performance on multiple domains of cognitive function. Cognitive deficits may occur at the very earliest stages of diabetes and are further exacerbated by the metabolic syndrome. The duration of diabetes and glycemic control may have an impact on the cognitive impairment. T2DM is more strongly associated with dementia as compared to T1DM. Various cognitive functions like impaired attention, processing and motor speed, executive functioning, and verbal memory are affected. Diabetes mellitus is a significant risk factor for not only vascular dementia, but AD as well. Diabetic patients have an approximately 60% increased risk of dementia. There is a 40% risk of nonvascular dementia. The pathophysiology of diabetic cognitive impairment is complex but is likely to involve impaired insulin signalling, increased inflammatory and oxidative stress pathways, and defects in mitochondrial metabolism and regulation. Both structural and functional abnormalities can be diagnosed by MRI/fMRI and MRS in diabetic patients. Cognitive impairment is associated with deficits in diabetes self-care behaviours, including poor compliance with medication, diet, and exercise recommendations, failure to receive appropriate care, and worse glycemic control including more hypoglycemia/hyperglycemia and further deterioration of cognitive function. In T2DM, lifestyle interventions that couple aerobic exercise with tailored dietary interventions currently offer the most likely benefit. Other therapies that improve insulin signalling or sensitivity may also offer benefit and trials with GLP-1 mimetics are currently active. Other therapies including anti-oxidants and anti-inflammatory medications have shown effectiveness in animal models.

Conclusion: Diabetes mellitus is associated with cognitive impairment. Pathophysiology is complex but it depends on duration and glycemic control. Frequent hypo and hyperglycemia, common in patients with cognitive impairment, are associated with decline in the cognitive functions.

100. Diabetes Medicines and Oral Health – Focus on Metformin and SGLT2i

S Sengupta

ABSTRACT

Diabetes affects multiple organ systems, including the oral cavity. Poor glycaemic control increases the risk of periodontal disease. Hyperglycaemia contributes to dry mouth (xerostomia) and increased infection risk. Delayed wound healing in diabetics affects oral tissues. Medications play a crucial role in modulating oral health outcomes.

Metformin is considered to be a first-line therapy for type 2 diabetes. Primarily reduces hepatic glucose production. Improves insulin sensitivity and reduces intestinal glucose absorption. Has anti-inflammatory and potential microbiome-modulating effects. Long-term use is associated with vitamin B12 deficiency. May impact oral and dental health through systemic effects.

Metformin has potential anti-inflammatory effects on gum tissues. May reduce gingival inflammation and periodontal pocket depth. Improves insulin resistance, indirectly benefiting oral tissues. Lowers oxidative stress, aiding in periodontal healing. Reduces levels of inflammatory cytokines like TNF-α and IL-6. Could have a protective role in preventing periodontitis progression.

SGLT2i includes empagliflozin, dapagliflozin, and canagliflozin. Promotes glucose excretion via urine by inhibiting sodium-glucose cotransporters. Benefits include weight loss, blood pressure reduction, and cardiovascular protection. Increases urinary glucose, which may impact microbial flora. Reduces insulin levels, potentially altering oral tissue responses. SGLT2i reduces systemic inflammation, potentially benefiting gum health. May help in reducing periodontal pocket depth. Indirect benefits through improved glycemic control and weight loss. SGLT2i prevents reabsorption of glucose in the kidneys, and thereby increases urinary glucose excretion (i.e., glycosuria). This could lead to dehydration and increased thirst. Both associated with oral dryness (xerostomia). When undergoing dental procedures that may involve reduced food intake, patients on SGLT2is should consult their doctor about potential **increased risk of diabetic ketoacidosis** and may need to temporarily stop their medication.

Follow up: Encourage regular dental visits every 6 months. Maintain good glycemic control for optimal oral health. Use saliva substitutes or stimulants for xerostomia. Reinforce proper brushing and flossing techniques. Educate patients on recognizing early symptoms of oral infections.

101. Advancements in Renal Protection: Insights from Key Clinical Trials in CKD and Type 2 Diabetes

Arvind Gupta

ABSTRACT

CKD is a progressive disorder characterized by persistent kidney damage and reduced glomerular filtration rate (GFR), leading to increased cardiovascular and all-cause mortality. In patients with T2D, the risk of CKD progression is significantly amplified due to chronic hyperglycemia, hypertension, and inflammation. Traditional management approaches, including renin-angiotensin-aldosterone system (RAAS) inhibition and glycemic control, have provided partial renoprotection but have not fully halted disease progression. Recent large-scale clinical trials have introduced novel therapeutic strategies that offer superior renal outcomes. This review highlights key clinical trials that have shaped contemporary treatment paradigms, focusing on sodium-glucose cotransporter-2 (SGLT2) inhibitors, mineralocorticoid receptor antagonists (MRAs), and glucagon-like peptide-1 receptor agonists (GLP-1 RAs), among other emerging therapies.

- *CREDENCE Trial*: Canagliflozin significantly reduced the risk of major cardiovascular events (HR: 0.80, 95% CI: 0.67–0.95, $p = 0.01$), with similar benefits observed in both primary (HR: 0.68, 95% CI: 0.49-0.94) and secondary (HR: 0.85, 95% CI: 0.69–1.06) prevention groups. Cardiovascular death (HR: 0.78), nonfatal myocardial infarction (HR: 0.81), and nonfatal stroke (HR: 0.80) were consistently reduced. Renal outcomes and cardiovascular death or hospitalization for heart failure were also favorably impacted ($p > 0.5$ for interaction).
- *DAPA-CKD Trial*: Dapagliflozin 10 mg/day was tested in patients with CKD (eGFR 25–75 mL/min/1.73 m^2, UACR ≥200 mg/g). The primary endpoint was a composite of ≥50% eGFR decline, ESKD, renal death, or cardiovascular death. The trial aimed for 90% power to detect a 22% relative risk reduction with 681 primary renal events.
- *FIDELIO-DKD Trial*: Finerenone reduced the composite cardiovascular outcome (CV death, MI, stroke, HF hospitalization) in CKD and T2D patients regardless of heart failure history (HR: 0.73 with HF, HR: 0.90 without HF, p for interaction = 0.33). The kidney composite outcome (kidney failure, ≥40% eGFR decline, or renal death) showed consistent benefits (HR: 0.79 with HF, HR: 0.83 without HF, p for interaction = 0.83).
- *FIGARO-DKD Trial*: Finerenone showed a trend toward kidney protection (HR: 0.87, $p = 0.069$) and significantly reduced ≥57% eGFR decline (HR: 0.77, $p = 0.041$). A 36% relative risk reduction for ESKD was observed. Benefits were greater in patients with severely increased albuminuria.
- *EMPA-KIDNEY Trial*: Empagliflozin reduced kidney disease progression or cardiovascular death (HR: 0.72, 95% CI: 0.64–0.82, $p < 0.001$) over a median 2-year follow-up. Benefits were consistent across eGFR subgroups and in both diabetic and non-diabetic patients. Hospitalization risk was lower (HR: 0.86, $p = 0.003$), but no significant differences were seen for heart failure hospitalization or all-cause mortality.
- *CANVAS Program*: Canagliflozin significantly reduced the risk of kidney disease progression (HR: 0.53, 95% CI: 0.33–0.84) and slowed eGFR decline (1.2 mL/min/1.73 m^2 per year difference). Mean UACR was 18% lower with canagliflozin. Renal-related adverse events were similar between groups (HR: 0.76, 95% CI: 0.49–1.19).
- *LEADER Trial*: Liraglutide reduced major cardiovascular events (HR: 0.87, $p < 0.001$ for noninferiority, $p = 0.01$ for superiority) and cardiovascular death (HR: 0.78, $p = 0.007$). All-cause mortality was also lower (HR: 0.85, $p = 0.02$). The incidence of nonfatal MI, stroke, and HF hospitalization was lower but not statistically significant.

- *REWIND Trial*: Dulaglutide reduced major cardiovascular events (HR: 0.88, $p = 0.026$) over a median 5.4-year follow-up. All-cause mortality was similar between groups ($p = 0.067$). Gastrointestinal adverse events were significantly more frequent with dulaglutide ($p < 0.0001$).
- *FLOW Trial*: In patients with CKD and T2D, once-weekly subcutaneous semaglutide significantly improved renal and cardiovascular outcomes over a median follow-up of 3.4 years. It reduced all-cause and cardiovascular mortality across various CKD severities. Additional benefits included a modest reduction in body weight (4.1 kg), HbA1c (0.81%), and systolic BP (2.2 mm Hg). Semaglutide also slowed eGFR decline by 1.16 mL/min/1.73 m^2, marking a major advancement in CKD and T2D management.

These findings underscore the transformative role of SGLT2 inhibitors, MRAs, and GLP-1 receptor agonists in CKD management among patients with T2D. Future research should explore combination therapies and long-term impacts on renal and cardiovascular health.

102. Acute Complications of Diabetes

Ahmed Al-Sharefi

ABSTRACT

Topic 1: Acute complications of diabetes

Session overview: The session will discuss hyperglycaemic crises such as diabetes ketoacidosis, hyperosmolar hyperglycaemia state and also hypoglycaemia. We will also discuss possible complications that may arise from treating these complications and how to avoid them. By the end of the session, attendants will be able to recognise the wide spectrum of presentations accompanying diabetic emergencies and gain confidence in approaching them safely and effectively.

Topic 2: Reproductive and sexual health for patients with diabetes

Session overview: Sex is a vital component of the emotional and relational fabric within couples and families. As the prevalence of diabetes continues to rise, it increasingly influences sexual and reproductive health, often in ways that go unaddressed. Many individuals—both men and women—who attend diabetes clinics may hesitate to disclose the impact of their condition on sexual and reproductive well-being due to the sensitive nature of the topic, feelings of embarrassment, or a lack of awareness regarding these complications. In this session, we will explore the relationship between diabetes, its treatment, and sexual health for couples. We will discuss practical strategies that healthcare providers can implement to address these challenges, fostering open communication and enhancing patient.

103. Oral Microbiome in Patients with Diabetes: Recent Insights

Chandni Radhakrishnan, Rosamma Joseph

ABSTRACT

The bidirectional relationship between diabetes and the oral microbiome is gaining importance in understanding the link between oral health and metabolic disorders like diabetes.

Diabetes, particularly poorly controlled type 2 diabetes, is associated with significant alterations in the oral microbiome characterised by higher concentrations of pathogenic bacteria connected to periodontal disease. Elevated blood glucose in saliva creates a more favourable environment for the growth of bacteria in the mouth heightening the risk of oral infections such as periodontal disease. Chronic inflammation of diabetes also contributes to dysbiosis in the oral cavity. Inflammatory cytokines linked to diabetes can modify the oral environment, making it more conducive to the growth of pathogenic bacteria.

In individuals with diabetes, periodontal disease is more common and more severe. The presence of periodontal pathogens can exacerbate the systemic inflammation associated with diabetes, potentially worsening insulin resistance and contributing to poor glycaemic control. The oral cavity harbours a large number of bacteria, and some of these bacteria can enter the bloodstream through gingival tissues, particularly in the presence of periodontal disease. These bacteria, along with their endotoxins, can lead to systemic inflammation, which may impair insulin sensitivity and increase the risk of developing or worsening diabetes.

Recent studies have shown that specific microbial signatures in the oral microbiome could serve as biomarkers for early detection and assessing the risk of developing diabetes. Advances in metabolomics have revealed that the metabolic byproducts of oral bacteria, such as short-chain fatty acids, may directly impact systemic metabolic health. Probiotic therapies or the use of oral antibacterials to control pathogenic bacteria have shown promise in improving both oral and metabolic health. Improving oral hygiene in individuals with diabetes leads to better glycemic control by reducing inflammation and bacterial load in the mouth.

There is growing potential for personalised approaches to treat diabetes based on an individual's unique oral microbiome with tailored interventions to improve systemic health. Future research for microbiome-based diagnostic tools predicting diabetes progression and complications will open up new avenues for potential interventions.